CLINICAL ENGLISH ESSENTIALS FOR NURSES

BRIDGING LANGUAGE AND HEALTHCARE

Dr. Alaric Naudé

Clinical English Essentials for Nurses: BRIDGING LANGUAGE AND HEALTHCARE

 Editing and Typesetting by Lindsey Crow

ISBN: 978-1-7637811-4-6

Dedication

To my students who have helped me learn a lot over the many years of teaching and letting me use them as test subjects for new ideas.

Contents

Chapter 1: The Significance of Greek and Latin Roots in Medical Terminology and Anatomy

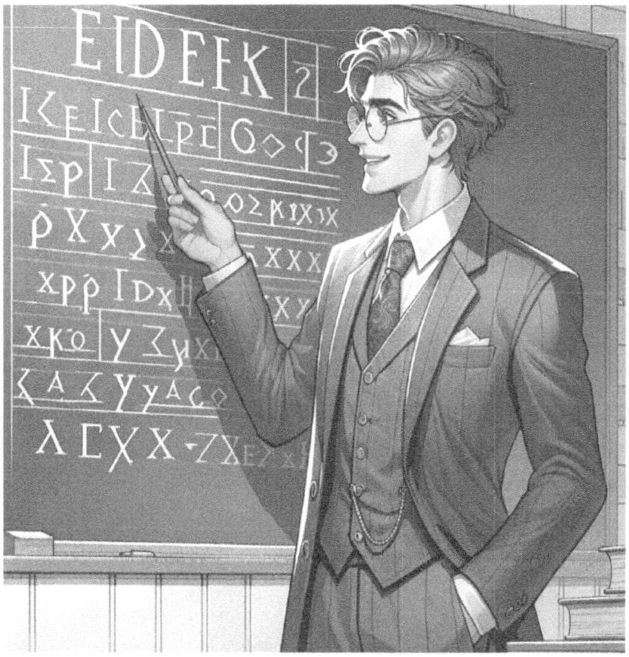

Understanding medical terminology and anatomy often involves delving into the origins of words, many of which are derived from Greek and Latin. These languages form the foundation of much of the medical vocabulary, with roots, prefixes, and suffixes acting like building blocks to create new words. By learning these components, students can more easily understand and remember medical terms.

Greek and Latin Roots: The Building Blocks

In medical terminology, Greek and Latin words come together to form complex terms. This is similar to how 'biology' is formed from 'bio-' (life) and '-ology' (study of). Instead of memorizing full words, understanding individual parts makes it easier to grasp the meaning of new terms. For instance, 'biologist' combines 'bio-' (life) and '-ologist' (person who studies).

Key Medical Terms and Their Origins

1. **Ophthalmology (ὀφθαλμός)**: 'Ophthalmo-' (eye) + '-logy' (study of). The branch of medicine dealing with the eyes.
2. **Ophthalmologist**: 'Ophthalmo-' (eye) + '-ologist' (person who studies). A specialist in ophthalmology.
3. **Dentistry**: 'Dent-' (tooth) + '-istry' (practice of). The branch of medicine concerned with the study, diagnosis, and treatment of oral conditions.
4. **Dentist**: 'Dent-' (tooth) + '-ist' (specialist). A practitioner of dentistry.
5. **Orthopaedics**: 'Ortho-' (straight) + 'paedia' (child). The branch of medicine dealing with the correction of deformities of bones or muscles.

6. **Paediatrics**: 'Paedia' (child) + '-iatrics' (medical practice). The branch of medicine dealing with children and their diseases.
7. **Radiology**: 'Radio-' (radiation) + '-logy' (study of). The science dealing with X-rays and other high-energy radiation.
8. **Obstetrics**: From the Latin 'obstetrix' (midwife). The branch of medicine concerned with childbirth and the care of women giving birth.
9. **Gynaecology (γυναικολογία)**: 'Gynae-' (woman) + '-logy' (study of). The branch of medicine dealing with the health of the female reproductive system.
10. **Pathology (παθολογία)**: 'Patho-' (disease) + '-logy' (study of). The study of the causes and effects of diseases.
11. **Dermatology (δερματολογία)**: 'Dermato-' (skin) + '-logy' (study of). The branch of medicine dealing with the skin.
12. **Oncology (ὀγκολογία)**: 'Onco-' (tumor) + '-logy' (study of). The branch of medicine dealing with tumors.
13. **Urology (ουρολογία)**: 'Uro-' (urine) + '-logy' (study of). The branch of medicine dealing with the urinary system.
14. **Otorhinolaryngology**: 'Oto-' (ear) + 'rhino-' (nose) + 'laryngo-' (throat) + '-logy' (study of). The study of diseases of the ear, nose, and throat.
15. **Neurology (νευρολογία)**: 'Neuro-' (nerve) + '-logy' (study of). The branch of medicine dealing with disorders of the nervous system.
16. **Neurosurgery**: 'Neuro-' (nerve) + 'surgery'. The surgical specialty involving the nervous system.
17. **General Practitioner**: A medical doctor who is trained to provide primary healthcare to patients of all ages.
18. **Hospice**: From the Latin 'hospitium' (hospitality). A type of care focusing on the palliation of a terminally ill patient's symptoms.
19. **Geriatrics**: From the Greek 'geras' (old age) + '-iatrics' (medical practice). The branch of medicine focusing on health and care of elderly people.

By familiarizing themselves with these roots, students and professionals in the medical field can gain a deeper understanding of the language of medicine. This approach not only aids in memorization but also enhances the comprehension of complex medical concepts.

TASK 1: FILL IN THE BLANKS

1. **Ophthalmology** is the study of the ____, derived from the Greek word 'ὀφθαλμός'.
2. A **Dentist** is a specialist in ________, which involves the study and treatment of teeth.
3. **Orthopaedics** deals with correcting deformities in bones or muscles, with 'Ortho-' meaning ______ and 'paedia' meaning _____.
4. The branch of medicine focusing on children and their diseases is called _________.
5. **Radiology** involves the study of ________ and is derived from 'Radio-'.
6. **Obstetrics** is concerned with ________ and the care of women during this process.
7. **Gynaecology**, from the Greek 'γυναικολογία', deals with the health of the ______ reproductive system.
8. **Pathology**, or 'παθολογία' in Greek, is the study of _______ and their effects.

9. A practitioner in **Dermatology** specializes in treating conditions related to the ______.
10. **Oncology**, derived from 'ὀγκολογία', is the branch of medicine that deals with _______.
11. **Urology** is the study of the urinary system, with 'Uro-' referring to ______.
12. **Neurology** focuses on disorders of the ______ system.
13. A **General Practitioner** is a medical doctor who provides _______ healthcare.
14. **Hospice** care, focusing on terminally ill patients, derives its name from the Latin word for _______.
15. **Geriatrics** involves the care of ________ people, with 'Geras' meaning old age in Greek.

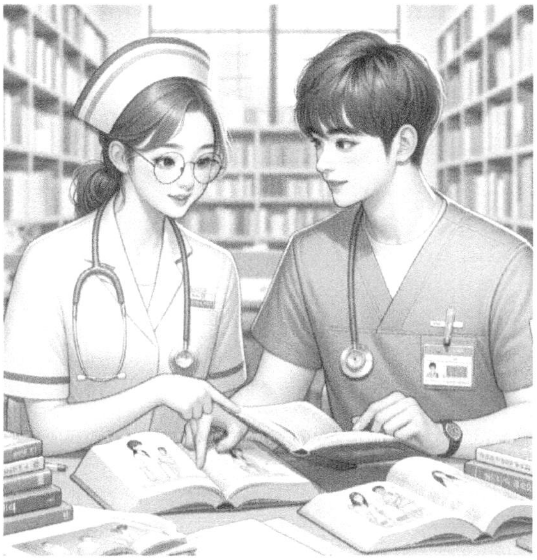

TASK 2: LET'S TALK

Mia: Hey Ethan, did you go through Professor Johnson's lecture notes on Greek and Latin roots in medical terminology?

Ethan: Yeah, I did. I was actually surprised at how much easier it made understanding these complex medical terms.

Mia: Right? I always thought it was about memorizing long, complicated words. But breaking them down into parts makes so much more sense. Like how 'ophthalmology' is all about the study of the eye.

Ethan: Exactly! And take 'dentistry' for instance. Knowing that 'dent-' means tooth simplifies things a lot. It's the same with 'dentist'. It's all about treating teeth.

Mia: The one on 'orthopaedics' was interesting too. 'Ortho-' meaning straight and 'paedia' meaning child. It paints a clear picture of what that field deals with.

Ethan: I was intrigued by 'paediatrics'. It's all about children's medical care, and the term literally means that.

Mia: And how about 'radiology'? It's just the study of radiation. Professor Johnson really did a great job of simplifying these terms.

Ethan: 'Obstetrics' and 'gynaecology' were eye-openers too. I never knew that obstetrics was related to childbirth, and gynaecology is all about women's reproductive health.

Mia: The lecture on 'pathology' was my favorite. It's the study of diseases, and knowing that 'patho-' means disease makes it so much clearer.

Ethan: It's the same with 'dermatology' and 'oncology'. Skin and tumors, respectively. Once you know the root, the rest follows.

Mia: Did you catch the bit about 'urology'? It's literally the study of urine. Makes me realize how logical these terms are.

Ethan: Yeah, and 'neurology' too. It's all about the nervous system. 'Neuro-' refers to nerves. It's fascinating how these terms are built.

Mia: This approach is going to make studying for our exams so much easier. I'm glad Professor Johnson emphasized this method.

Ethan: Definitely. It's not just rote memorization anymore. It's about understanding the language of medicine.

TASK 3: DO YOU REMEMBER?

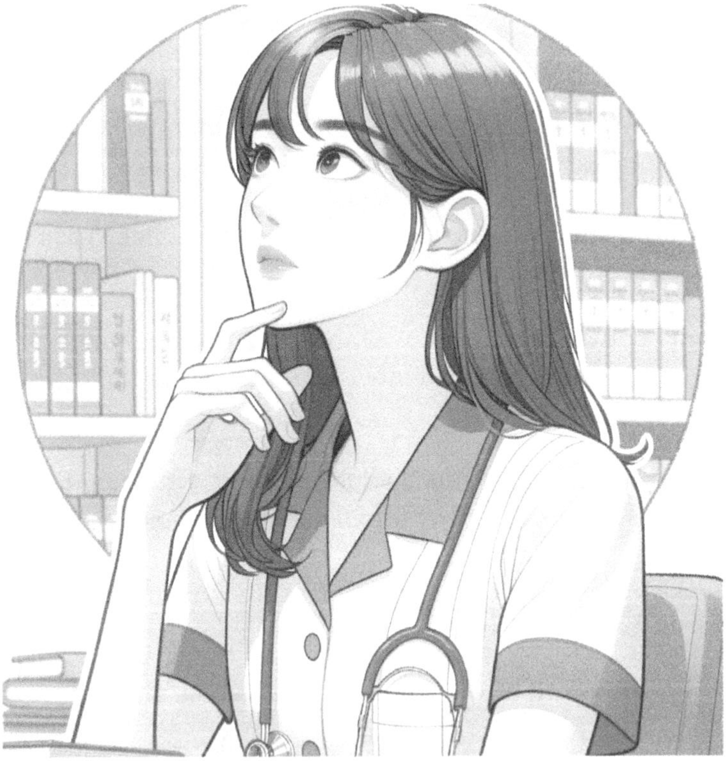

1. **What does the root 'ophthalmo-' in 'ophthalmology' refer to?**

2. **In the term 'dentistry', what does the root 'dent-' mean?**

3. **What are the meanings of 'Ortho-' and 'paedia' in the term 'orthopaedics'?**

4. **What medical field does 'paediatrics' relate to, and what does the term mean?**

5. **From which root does 'radiology' derive its meaning, and what does it study?**

6. **What aspect of women's health does 'gynaecology' focus on?**

7. **In the term 'pathology', what does 'patho-' signify?**

8. **What is the focus area of 'dermatology', based on its Greek root?**

9. **'Oncology' deals with the study of what?**

10. **How does the term 'urology' relate to its Greek origin, and what does it study?**

TASK 4: MAKE A CHOICE

1. What does ophthalmology primarily deal with?

   A) Bones B) Eyes C) Ears D) Teeth

2. Who is a specialist in ophthalmology?

   A) Orthopedist B) Ophthalmologist

   C) Dermatologist D) Oncologist

3. What is the focus of dentistry?

A) Eye conditions B) Bone deformities

C) Oral conditions D) Skin conditions

4. What is a dentist specialized in?

   A) Child healthcare B) Tooth and oral care

   C) Radiation therapy D) Women's health

5. What does orthopaedics primarily deal with?

   A) Urinary systems B) Eye disorders

   C) Correction of bone deformities D) Childbirth

6. Paediatrics is a branch of medicine dealing with:

   A) Tumors

   B) Children and their diseases

   C) Nervous system disorders

   D) Ear, nose, and throat diseases

7. What does radiology involve?

   A) Child healthcare B) Radiation and X-rays

   C) Dental treatments D) Bone surgery

8. Obstetrics is concerned with:

   A) Female reproductive health

   B) Childbirth and care of pregnant women

   C) Urinary disorders

D) Skin diseases

9. Gynaecology deals with:

A) Diseases of the ear, nose, and throat

B) Health of the female reproductive system

C) Dental health

D) Bone and muscle deformities

10. What is the focus of pathology?

A) The study of radiation

B) Causes and effects of diseases

C) Old age health issues

D) Nervous system surgeries

11. Dermatology is the branch of medicine dealing with:

A) The skin B) The eyes

C) Child health D) Bones and muscles

12. What does oncology focus on?

A) Urinary system disorders B) Tumors and cancers

C) Dental diseases D) Old age health care

13. Urology is a branch of medicine that deals with:

A) The urinary system B) Childbirth

C) Nerve disorders D) Ear, nose, and throat

14. What does otorhinolaryngology study?

A) Diseases of the ear, nose, and throat

B) Eye disorders

C) Urinary system disorders

D) Tumor

15. What is neurology concerned with?

A) Bone surgeries B) Disorders of the nervous system

C) Dental health D) Radiology

Chapter 2: Nursing Equipment

Nurses rely on a variety of medical equipment to provide patient care efficiently and effectively. Each tool, whether simple or sophisticated, serves a specific purpose in the assessment, diagnosis, and treatment of patients. This guide delves into the details of these essential tools, including the various types of medical gloves used in healthcare settings.

STETHOSCOPE

The stethoscope, an acoustic device, is used for auscultation, or listening to the internal sounds of the body. It typically consists of a small resonator that's placed against the chest and two tubes connected to earpieces. Nurses use stethoscopes to listen to heartbeats, lung sounds, and bowel activity. Electronic stethoscopes are also available, which amplify these sounds for a more detailed analysis.

SPHYGMOMANOMETER

A sphygmomanometer, or blood pressure cuff, measures arterial blood pressure. It comprises an inflatable cuff to restrict blood flow and a mercury or aneroid manometer to measure the pressure. Manual sphygmomanometers are used with a stethoscope, while digital models provide automatic measurements.

THERMOMETER

Thermometers measure body temperature and come in various forms:

- **Digital Thermometers**: Provide quick and accurate readings orally, rectally, or under the armpit.
- **Ear (Tympanic) Thermometers**: Measure temperature from the ear and are less invasive.
- **Infrared Thermometers**: Allow for non-contact temperature measurement, ideal for infection control.

PULSE OXIMETER

This small device clips onto a patient's finger, toe, or earlobe to measure the oxygen saturation level of the blood. It's essential for patients undergoing anaesthesia, in intensive care, or with respiratory issues.

GLUCOMETER

Glucometers are used to measure the concentration of glucose in the blood. They are vital for diabetes management, requiring only a small blood sample placed on a test strip.

ECG MACHINE

The Electrocardiogram (ECG) machine records the heart's electrical activity over time. It helps diagnose arrhythmias, myocardial infarction, and other cardiac conditions. Portable ECG monitors are also available for ambulatory use.

IV PUMPS

Intravenous (IV) pumps administer fluids, blood, or medications directly into the bloodstream at controlled rates. They are crucial in maintaining accurate dosing and ensuring patient safety.

NEBULIZERS

Nebulizers are essential for delivering medication directly to the lungs in an aerosol form. They are especially useful in treating asthma, COPD, and other respiratory conditions.

DEFIBRILLATORS

Defibrillators deliver a therapeutic dose of electric current to the heart. Automated External Defibrillators (AEDs) are commonly found in public spaces for emergency use.

PATIENT MONITORING SYSTEMS

These systems continuously monitor vital signs like ECG, blood pressure, oxygen saturation, and respiratory rate. They are indispensable in critical care environments for real-time patient assessment.

SYRINGES AND NEEDLES

Syringes and needles are fundamental for administering injections or withdrawing bodily fluids. They vary in size and type, including insulin syringes, tuberculin syringes, and hypodermic syringes.

OTOSCOPE

An otoscope is used to examine the external auditory canal and tympanic membrane. It comprises a light source and a magnifying lens for detailed examination.

OPHTHALMOSCOPE

This device enables the examination of the interior structures of the eye. It's particularly important for diagnosing diseases of the retina and optic nerve.

MEDICAL SCALES

Medical scales, including digital and mechanical types, accurately measure a patient's weight. Bariatric scales are available for heavier patients, and infant scales are used for newborns.

MEDICAL GLOVES

Medical gloves are crucial for infection control. They come in different types:

- **Latex Gloves**: Offer high tactile sensitivity, flexibility, and comfort.

- **Nitrile Gloves**: Latex-free, these are suitable for those with latex allergies and provide excellent resistance to chemicals and punctures.

- **Nitrile Gloves**: Latex-free, these are suitable for those with latex allergies and provide excellent resistance to chemicals and punctures.

- **Neoprene Gloves**: Offer excellent flexibility and chemical resistance, suitable for surgical procedures.

The array of medical equipment used in nursing is diverse, each serving a specific purpose in patient care. From basic tools like thermometers to advanced machines like ECGs, and including various types of medical gloves, these tools are essential for nurses to perform their roles effectively and safely. Understanding and efficiently using this equipment is fundamental in the nursing profession, ensuring high standards of patient care and safety.

TASK 1: FILL IN THE BLANKS

1. A _________ is used by nurses to listen to internal sounds of the body like heartbeats and lung sounds.
2. Blood pressure is measured using a ____________, which consists of an inflatable cuff and a pressure measuring device.
3. To measure body temperature, nurses often use a ___________, which can be digital, tympanic, or ________.
4. A ___________ is a device that measures the oxygen saturation level in the blood by attaching to a patient's ________.
5. Nurses use ___________ to monitor blood glucose levels, especially in patients with diabetes.
6. An _______ machine records the heart's electrical activity and is crucial in diagnosing _________ conditions.
7. An _______ machine records the heart's electrical activity and is crucial in diagnosing _________ conditions.
8. Medications for respiratory conditions like asthma are often administered using a ___________.
9. In emergency situations, a ___________ is used to deliver an electric shock to the heart.
10. Vital signs like blood pressure and heart rate are continuously monitored using ___________ systems.
11. Nurses use different types of __________ and needles for administering injections or drawing fluids.

12. An _________ is employed to examine the ears, while an ___________ is used for eye examinations.

13. ___________ are essential for accurate weight measurement in a healthcare setting.

14. Nurses wear ________ gloves for infection control, which can be made of latex, ________, vinyl, or neoprene.

15. ________ gloves are preferred for individuals with latex allergies and provide resistance to chemicals and punctures.

TASK 2: LET'S TALK

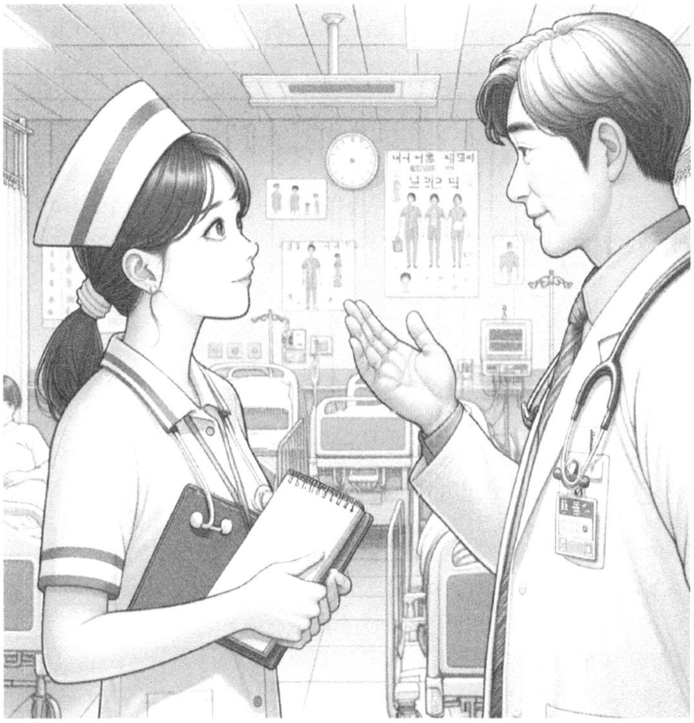

Sarah: Hi James, I'm still getting familiar with where everything is. Could you help me understand where to find some of the medical supplies and machines we use daily?

James: Of course, Sarah. What are you looking for first?

Sarah: Where do we keep the stethoscopes?

James: We have a supply of stethoscopes in each nurse's station. You'll find them hanging on the hooks near the blood pressure monitors.

Sarah: Speaking of blood pressure monitors, where are the sphygmomanometers stored?

James: They're usually right next to the stethoscopes. We have both manual and digital ones. The manual ones are in the top drawer, and the digital ones are on the shelf above.

Sarah: Got it. And the thermometers?

James: For digital and tympanic thermometers, check the small cabinets in each examination room. Infrared thermometers are in the isolation rooms and at the front desk for quick checks.

Sarah: What about pulse oximeters?

James: Those are kept in the central supply room. You'll find them in the drawer labeled 'Respiratory Equipment.'

Sarah: I also need to find glucometers for diabetic patients.

James: The glucometers are in the diabetes care section of the supply room. Right next to the glucometers, you'll find the test strips and lancets.

Sarah: And if I need an ECG machine?

James: The portable ECG machines are in the cardiology department. But for immediate use, we have one in each emergency response cart.

Sarah: Where do we store IV pumps?

James: IV pumps are on the medication carts. If you need more, there are extras in the equipment storage room.

Sarah: I'm also supposed to administer a nebulizer treatment today.

James: Nebulizers are in the respiratory therapy room. Make sure to check if the medication chamber and masks are attached.

Sarah: If a situation calls for a defibrillator?

James: There's an AED located in every hallway and major patient area. For advanced defibrillators, check the emergency response carts.

Sarah: Lastly, where can I find the different types of medical gloves?

James: We have glove dispensers throughout the hospital. The dispensers usually have labels indicating whether they're latex, nitrile, or vinyl. Neoprene gloves are usually reserved for surgical procedures, so they're in the OR supply room.

Sarah: Thanks so much, James. This really helps!

James: No problem, Sarah. You'll get the hang of it soon. If you need anything else, just ask.

TASK 3: DO YOU REMEMBER?

1. **Where are stethoscopes commonly stored in a hospital?**

2. **What types of sphygmomanometers can be found near the nurse's station?**

3. **Where are digital and tympanic thermometers usually kept?**

4. **In which rooms are infrared thermometers primarily located?**

5. **Where can a nurse find pulse oximeters in the hospital?**

6. **In which section of the supply room are glucometers stored?**

7. **Where does one find portable ECG machines for immediate use?**

8. **Where are additional IV pumps stored besides the medication carts?**

9. **Where should a nurse go to find nebulizers and their components?**

10. **Where are Automated External Defibrillators (AEDs) located in the hospital?**

11. **What types of medical gloves are available in the glove dispensers throughout the hospital?**

12. **Where are neoprene gloves, typically used for surgical procedures, stored?**

13. **Which department stores the portable ECG machines for cardiological assessments?**

14. **Where in the hospital can a nurse find the emergency response carts?**

15. **What items are found in the drawer labelled 'Respiratory Equipment' in the central supply room?**

TASK 4: LATIN AND GREEK TIME

1. **Stethoscope**
   - *Stetho-* comes from the Greek word "stethos" (στῆθος), meaning chest.
   - *-scope* comes from the Greek word "skopein" (σκοπεῖν), meaning to look at or examine.
2. **Sphygmomanometer**
   - *Sphygmo-* comes from the Greek word "sphygmos" (σφυγμός), meaning pulse.
   - *-manometer* combines "manos" (μανός), meaning rare or sparse, and "metron" (μέτρον), meaning measure.
3. **Thermometer**
   - *Thermo-* comes from the Greek word "thermos" (θερμός), meaning hot.
   - *-meter* comes from the Greek word "metron" (μέτρον), meaning measure.
4. **Pulse Oximeter**
   - *Pulse* comes from the Latin word "pulsus," meaning beating or throbbing.
   - *Oxi-* comes from the Greek word "oxys" (ὀξύς), meaning sharp or acidic.

- *-meter* as above.

5. **Glucometer**

- *Gluco-* relates to glucose, from the Greek word "glykys" (γλυκύς), meaning sweet.
- *-meter* as above.

6. **Electrocardiogram (ECG)**

- *Electro-* comes from the Greek word "ēlektron" (ἤλεκτρον), meaning amber (referring to static electricity).
- *Cardio-* comes from the Greek word "kardia" (καρδιά), meaning heart.
- *-gram* comes from the Greek word "gramma" (γράμμα), meaning something written.

7. **Intravenous (IV)**

- *Intra-* comes from the Latin word "intra," meaning within.
- *Venous* comes from the Latin word "vena," meaning vein.

8. **Nebulizer**

- Derived from the Latin word "nebula," meaning mist or fog.

9. **Defibrillator**

- *De-* is a Latin prefix meaning away or from.
- *Fibrilla-* comes from the Latin word "fibrilla," meaning a small fiber.
- *-tor* is a Latin suffix indicating an agent or doer.

10. **Otoscope**

- *Oto-* comes from the Greek word "ous" (οὖς, genitive: ὠτός), meaning ear.
- *-scope* as above.

11. **Ophthalmoscope**

- *Ophthalmo-* as in stethoscope.
- *-scope* as above.

12. **Medical Scales**

- *Medical* comes from the Latin word "medicus," meaning physician.
- *Scales* comes from the Old Norse word "skal" (bowl, dish, scale), not directly from Latin or Greek.

13. **Medical Gloves**

- *Medical* as above.
- *Gloves* comes from the Old English word "glof," not directly from Latin or Greek.

14. **Neoprene Gloves**

- *Neo-* comes from the Greek word "neos" (νέος), meaning new.
- *Prene* is not directly from Latin or Greek, but relates to polychloroprene, a type of synthetic rubber.

15. **Vinyl Gloves**

- *Vinyl* comes from the Latin word "vinum," meaning wine, referring to the ethyl group in its structure.
- *Gloves* as above.

TASK 5: MAKE A CHOICE

1. What is a stethoscope primarily used for?

A) Measuring blood pressure

B) Listening to internal body sounds

C) Examining the eyes

D) Checking skin conditions

2. What does a sphygmomanometer measure?

A) Body temperature

B) Blood sugar levels

C) Arterial blood pressure

D) Oxygen saturation in the blood

3. Which of the following thermometers provides a non-contact method of measuring body temperature?

A) Digital Thermometers B) Ear Thermometers

C) Infrared Thermometers D) Mercury Thermometers

4. A pulse oximeter is used to measure:

A) Heart rate only

B) Blood pressure only

C) Oxygen saturation level of the blood

D) Glucose concentration in the blood

5. What is the main purpose of a glucometer?

A) Measuring blood pressure

B) Monitoring heart rate

C) Measuring the concentration of glucose in the blood

D) Determining oxygen levels

6. An ECG machine records:

A) Body temperature B) The heart's electrical activity

C) Blood glucose levels D) Blood oxygen saturation

7. What is the function of IV pumps?

A) To measure blood pressure

B) To deliver medication directly into the bloodstream

C) To check body temperature

D) To examine the ears

8. Nebulizers are primarily used for:

A) Delivering medication to the lungs

B) Monitoring heart activity

C) Measuring blood pressure

D) Checking ear health

9. What is the primary use of defibrillators?

A) To measure blood glucose

B) To deliver a dose of electric current to the heart

C) To administer medications

D) To monitor respiratory rate

10. Patient monitoring systems continuously track:

A) Weight and height

B) Vital signs like ECG and blood pressure

C) Glucose levels only

D) External body temperatures

Chapter 3: Brain anatomy

The human brain, a marvel of biological engineering, is an intricate organ responsible for our most complex functions. It's divided into several parts, each with unique responsibilities. This article provides a detailed overview of the cerebrum's lobes - the frontal, parietal, occipital, and temporal lobes - as well as the brainstem and cerebellum, highlighting their functions and associated conditions.

THE CEREBRUM: THE CENTER OF HIGHER BRAIN FUNCTION

The cerebrum, the largest part of the brain, is divided into four lobes, each responsible for different functions.

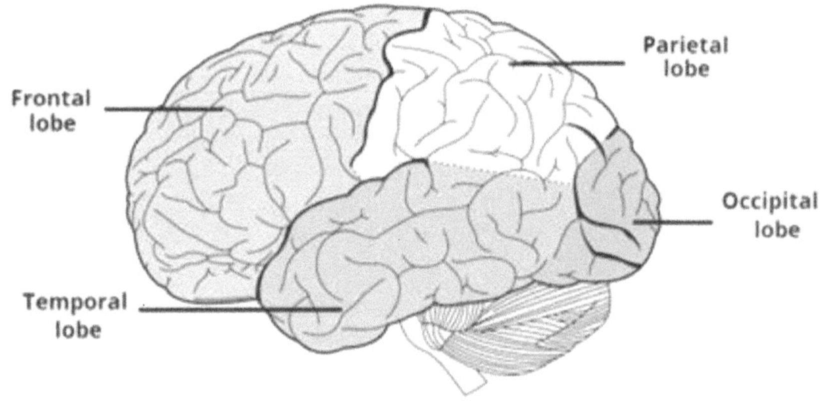

FRONTAL LOBE

- **Location and Function**: Situated at the front of the brain, the frontal lobe is associated with reasoning, motor skills, higher level cognition, and expressive language. It plays a crucial role in voluntary movement, managing higher emotions, and the ability to think abstractly.
- **Broca's Area**: Located in the frontal lobe, this region is critical for speech production. Damage to this area can result in Broca's aphasia, characterized by difficulties in speech production but relatively intact comprehension.
- **Associated Conditions**: Damage to the frontal lobe can lead to changes in personality, impaired judgment, and motor disorders. Conditions such as ADHD and schizophrenia are also linked to frontal lobe dysfunction.

PARIETAL LOBE

- **Location and Function**: Positioned behind the frontal lobe, the parietal lobe processes tactile sensory information like pressure, touch, and pain. It's significantly involved in processing spatial orientation and body awareness.
- **Somatosensory Cortex**: This area of the parietal lobe is vital for processing sensory information from various parts of the body.
- **Associated Conditions**: Issues in the parietal lobe can lead to problems with spatial reasoning, hand-eye coordination, and concentration. Dyscalculia, a difficulty in understanding numbers, can also arise.

OCCIPITAL LOBE

- **Location and Function**: The occipital lobe, located at the back of the brain, is primarily responsible for visual processing. It interprets information from the eyes, linking what we see with other parts of the brain.
- **Visual Disorders**: Damage to this area can cause visual disturbances such as difficulties recognizing objects or an inability to perceive motion.
- **Associated Conditions**: Conditions like cortical blindness, where eyes are functional but the brain cannot process visual stimuli, are linked to occipital lobe damage.

TEMPORAL LOBE

- **Location and Function**: Lying beneath the lateral fissure, the temporal lobe plays a role in processing auditory information and is essential in the understanding of language.
- **Wernicke's Area**: Found in the temporal lobe, this region is crucial for language comprehension. Wernicke's aphasia, resulting from damage to this area, leads to difficulties in understanding language.
- **Associated Conditions**: Problems in the temporal lobe can result in issues with memory, understanding language, sequencing, and organization. Disorders like Alzheimer's disease and dementia may have links to temporal lobe damage.

THE BRAINSTEM: LIFELINE OF THE BRAIN

The brainstem, located beneath the cerebrum and in front of the cerebellum, connects the brain to the spinal cord. It consists of three parts: the midbrain, pons, and medulla oblongata.

- **Functions**: The brainstem controls many basic life-sustaining functions, including heart rate, breathing, swallowing, and sleep cycles. It also plays a role in relaying information between the brain and the rest of the body.

- **Associated Conditions**: Damage to the brainstem can be life-threatening, affecting vital functions. Conditions like Locked-In Syndrome, where an individual is conscious but cannot move or communicate verbally due to complete paralysis, are associated with brainstem damage.

THE CEREBELLUM: THE BRAIN'S COORDINATOR

The cerebellum, located under the cerebrum at the back of the skull, plays a critical role in motor control.

- **Functions**: It does not initiate movement but contributes to coordination, precision, and accurate timing. It also plays a role in motor learning and maintaining posture and balance.

- **Associated Conditions**: Damage to the cerebellum can lead to ataxia, resulting in a lack of muscle control or coordination of voluntary movements. This can manifest as unsteady movements, clumsiness, or a disturbance in gait.

The brain, a complex and dynamic organ, orchestrates a wide range of functions through its different parts. The cerebrum, with its distinct lobes, manages everything from sensory processing and language to reasoning and movement. Meanwhile, the brainstem and cerebellum play essential roles in life-sustaining functions and motor control. Understanding the brain's anatomy and functions is fundamental to grasping how we interact with our environment, process thoughts and emotions, and perform daily.

TASK 1: FILL IN THE BLANKS

1. The __________ is divided into four lobes, each responsible for different functions.

2. The __________ lobe is linked with higher level cognition and motor skills.

3. In the frontal lobe, __________'s Area is vital for speech production.

4. The __________ lobe is involved in processing tactile sensations like touch and pressure.

5. The __________ cortex in the parietal lobe helps process sensory information from the body.

6. The __________ lobe is primarily tasked with visual information processing.

7. Auditory processing and language understanding are key functions of the __________ lobe.

8. Language comprehension issues, such as Wernicke's aphasia, are related to damage in the __________ lobe.

9. The __________ connects the brain to the spinal cord and manages basic life functions.

10. The __________ part of the brainstem plays a role in relaying information between the brain and body.

11. __________ is the part of the brain that aids in motor control and coordination.

12. Coordination problems like __________ can arise from damage to the cerebellum.

13. Difficulty in understanding numbers, known as dyscalculia, is linked to issues in the __________ lobe.

14. Problems with memory and organization may be due to damage in the __________ lobe.

15. The __________ lobe's dysfunction can lead to personality changes and impaired judgment.

TASK 2: LET'S TALK

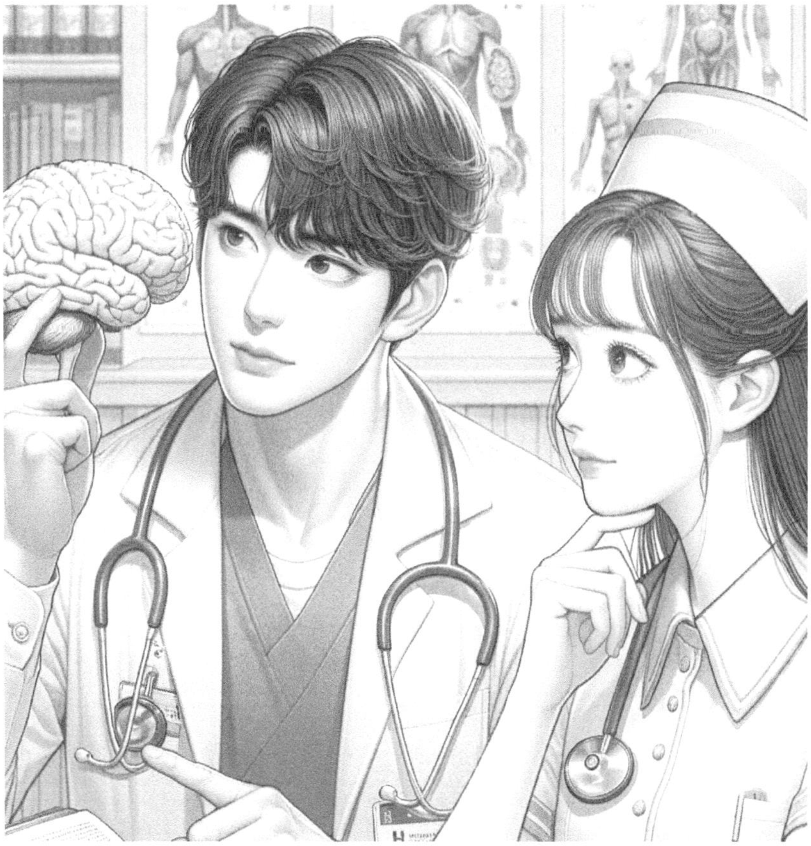

Emily: Okay, Liam, let's see if you can name the four lobes of the cerebrum without peeking at your notes!

Liam: Challenge accepted! There's the frontal lobe, parietal lobe, occipital lobe, and... umm... the temporal lobe!

Emily: Nice! Now, which one is responsible for our motor skills and higher level cognition?

Liam: That's easy, the frontal lobe. Our professor is so mean, making us study all these difficult things. I swear my own frontal lobe is going to explode!

Emily *(laughing)*: I know, right? But hey, what about the lobe that deals with sensory information like touch and pressure?

Liam: Oh, that's the parietal lobe. Speaking of pressure, I feel like my parietal lobe is under pressure with all this studying.

Emily: You're on a roll! Now, which lobe helps us process what we see?

Liam: That's the occipital lobe. Without it, we wouldn't be able to see the scowling face of our professor when we get these answers wrong!

Emily: True! And the temporal lobe, what does it do?

Liam: It's all about auditory processing and language comprehension. You know, I think our professor's temporal lobe is extra developed – he hears everything!

Emily: Haha, probably! Now, what about the part of the brain that connects to the spinal cord?

Liam: That's the brainstem. It's like the overseer of basic life functions. Maybe our professor is part brainstem, always keeping us in line!

Emily: Perfect! And lastly, the cerebellum?

Liam: Ah, the cerebellum, responsible for coordination and motor control. Maybe I need to exercise mine more to better coordinate my study schedule. Hahaha

Emily: Great job, Liam! We might just survive the professor's next pop quiz after all.

Liam: Thanks to our little game, I think we will. Now let's see if you can beat my score!

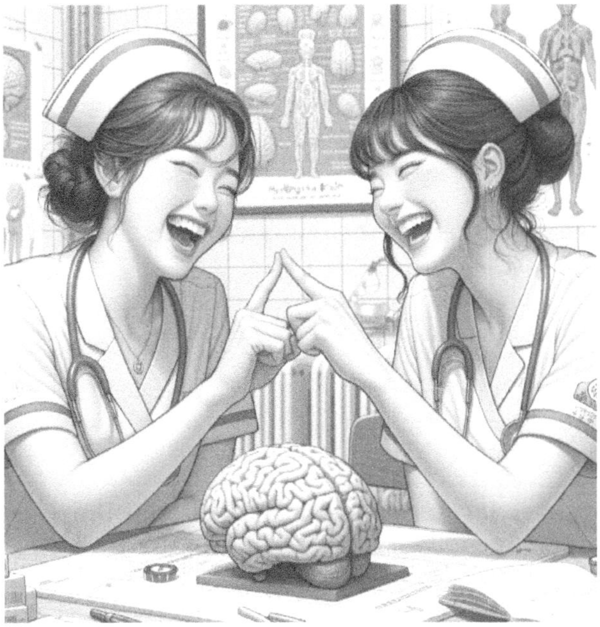

TASK 3: DO YOU REMEMBER?

1. **What are the four lobes of the cerebrum mentioned in the conversation?**

2. **Which lobe of the cerebrum is responsible for motor skills and higher level cognition?**

3. **What does the parietal lobe primarily process?**

4. **Which lobe is crucial for visual information processing?**

5. **What are the main functions of the temporal lobe as discussed by the students?**

6. **Where is Broca's area located, and what function is it associated with?**

7. **What condition might arise from damage to Wernicke's area in the temporal lobe?**

8. **What part of the brain connects the brain to the spinal cord?**

9. **Name one basic life function that the brainstem oversees.**

10. **What is the primary role of the cerebellum in the brain?**

11. **How does damage to the cerebellum manifest in terms of motor control?**

12. **What lobe is linked to issues with sensory information like touch and pressure?**

13. **Which lobe's dysfunction could lead to problems in understanding numbers?**

14. **What could be a consequence of damage to the frontal lobe in terms of personality?**

15. **According to the conversation, what humorous analogy do the students make about their professor and a part of the brain?**

TASK 4: LATIN AND GREEK TIME

1. **Cerebrum**

   - Comes from the Latin word "cerebrum," meaning brain.

2. **Frontal Lobe**

   - *Frontal* comes from the Latin word "frontalis," meaning of or belonging to the front.

3. **Parietal Lobe**

   - *Parietal* comes from the Latin word "parietalis," meaning of walls, relating to the walls of a cavity in the body.

4. **Occipital Lobe**

   - *Occipital* comes from the Latin word "occipitalis," pertaining to the occiput or the back of the head.

5. **Temporal Lobe**

   - *Temporal* comes from the Latin word "temporalis," meaning of the temples (sides of the head).

6. **Broca's Area**

   - Named after Paul Broca; the term itself does not have a Latin or Greek root.

7. **Aphasia**

   - Comes from the Greek word "aphasia" (ἀφασία), meaning speechlessness.

8. **Somatosensory Cortex**

   - *Somato-* comes from the Greek word "soma" (σῶμα), meaning body.
   - *Sensory* comes from the Latin word "sensōrius," meaning of or pertaining to the senses.
   - *Cortex* comes from the Latin word "cortex," meaning bark or outer layer.

9. **Dyscalculia**

   - *Dys-* comes from the Greek word "dys" (δυσ-), meaning bad or difficult.
   - *Calculia* comes from the Latin word "calculare," meaning to count.

10. **Cortical Blindness**

   - *Cortical* is derived from the Latin word "cortex," as above.
   - *Blindness* comes from the Old English word "blindnys," not directly from Latin or Greek.

11. **Wernicke's Area**

- Named after Carl Wernicke; the term itself does not have a Latin or Greek root.

12. **Brainstem**

- *Brain* comes from the Old English word "brægen," not directly from Latin or Greek
- *Stem* comes from the Old English word "stefn," "stæf," meaning stem, not directly from Latin or Greek.

13. **Cerebellum**

- Comes from the Latin word "cerebellum," meaning little brain.

14. **Ataxia**

- Comes from the Greek word "ataxia" (ἀταξία), meaning disorder or lack of order.

15. **Medulla Oblongata**

- *Medulla* comes from the Latin word "medulla," meaning marrow.
- *Oblongata* comes from the Latin word "oblongus," meaning more long than broad.

TASK 5: MAKE A CHOICE

1. What is the primary function of the cerebrum?

A) Motor control and coordination

B) Connecting the brain to the spinal cord

C) Higher brain functions like reasoning and language

D) Regulating basic life-sustaining functions

2. The frontal lobe is associated with:

A) Visual processing

B) Hearing and language comprehension

C) Motor skills and higher level cognition

D) Processing tactile sensory information

3. Broca's area, crucial for speech production, is located in the:

A) Temporal lobe B) Parietal lobe

C) Occipital lobe D) Frontal lobe

4. The parietal lobe primarily processes:

A) Sensory information like touch and pressure

B) Visual information

C) Language and speech

D) Emotions and abstract thinking

5. Which lobe is mainly responsible for visual processing?

A) Frontal lobe B) Parietal lobe

C) Occipital lobe D) Temporal lobe

6. The temporal lobe plays a key role in:

A) Processing auditory information

B) Movement coordination

C) Spatial reasoning

D) Heart rate control

7. Which area is vital for language comprehension?

A) Broca's area B) Wernicke's area

C) Somatosensory cortex D) Visual cortex

8. The brainstem is crucial for:

A) Intellectual functions B) Balance and posture

C) Basic life-sustaining functions D) Sensory processing

9. The cerebellum is primarily involved in:

A) Speech production B) Coordination and motor control

C) Vision and hearing D) Memory and learning

10. Damage to the occipital lobe can cause:

A) Speech disorders B) Visual disturbances

C) Loss of balance D) Impaired judgment

Chapter 4: Exploring Neurons and Glial Cells in the Nervous System

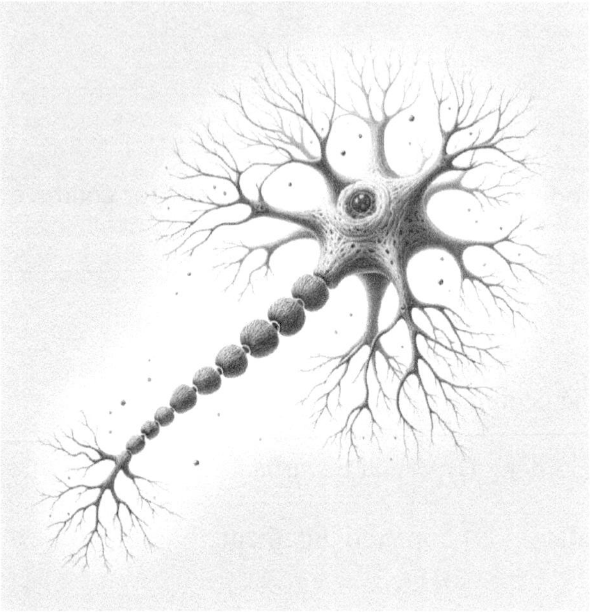

NEURONS: THE BRAIN'S MESSENGERS

Neurons are the primary cells in the brain and nervous system responsible for sending and receiving signals. These cells are incredibly numerous, with the cerebral cortex alone housing between 10 to 20 billion neurons and the cerebellum containing about 55 to 70 billion. They are the key players in transmitting information throughout the body.

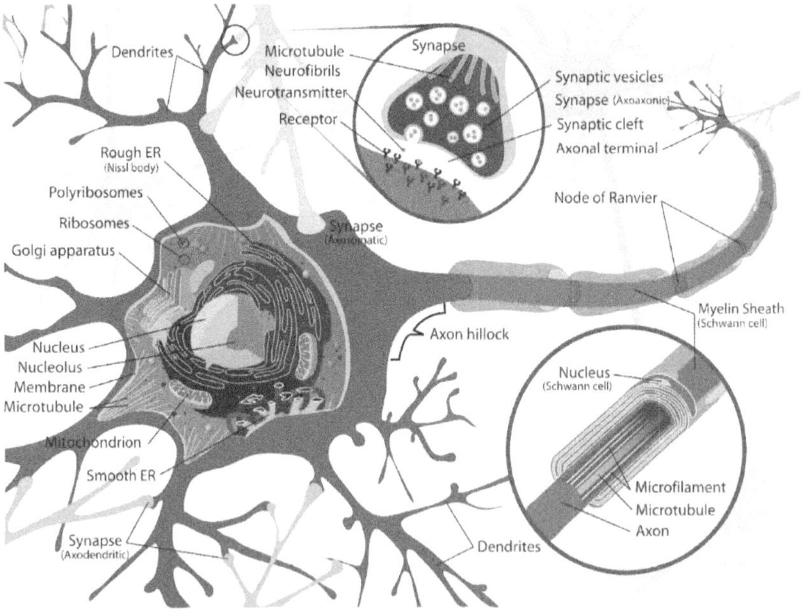

Neurons, often referred to as nerve cells, are the fundamental units of the brain and nervous system. They are responsible for transmitting information throughout the body. There are various types of neurons, each with specific structures and functions. Understanding these different types helps in grasping the complexity and efficiency of the human nervous system.

Types of Neurons

1. **Sensory Neurons (Afferent Neurons)**
    - **Function:** Sensory neurons are responsible for converting external stimuli from the environment into internal electrical impulses. For example, they help you sense heat, cold, pain, and other sensory stimuli.
    - **Structure:** They typically have a long dendrite and a short axon and are located in the sensory organs (like the skin) and the internal organs.
2. **Motor Neurons (Efferent Neurons)**
    - **Function:** Motor neurons transmit signals from the brain and spinal cord to the muscles and glands, thereby enabling movements and glandular responses.
    - **Structure:** These neurons have a long axon and short dendrites and connect to muscles, glands, and organs throughout the body.
3. **Interneurons (Association Neurons)**
    - **Function:** Interneurons are the most numerous neurons in the human nervous system. They connect sensory and motor neurons and carry out complex integrations and processing within the brain and spinal cord.
    - **Structure:** Interneurons have short axons and are found exclusively in the central nervous system (brain and spinal cord).

Subtypes of Neurons

In addition to these primary types, there are several subtypes of neurons based on their functions and locations:

1. **Pyramidal Cells**
    - Found in the cerebral cortex, pyramidal cells play a crucial role in cognitive functions such as planning and decision-making.
2. **Purkinje Cells**
    - Located in the cerebellum, these cells are essential for motor coordination and balance.
3. **Unipolar Neurons**
    - Typically sensory neurons with a single axon extending from the body, they are commonly found in the peripheral nervous system.

4. **Bipolar Neurons**

- Found in sensory pathways (like the retina of the eye), bipolar neurons have one axon and one dendrite.

SCHWANN CELLS: GUARDIANS OF THE PERIPHERAL NERVOUS SYSTEM

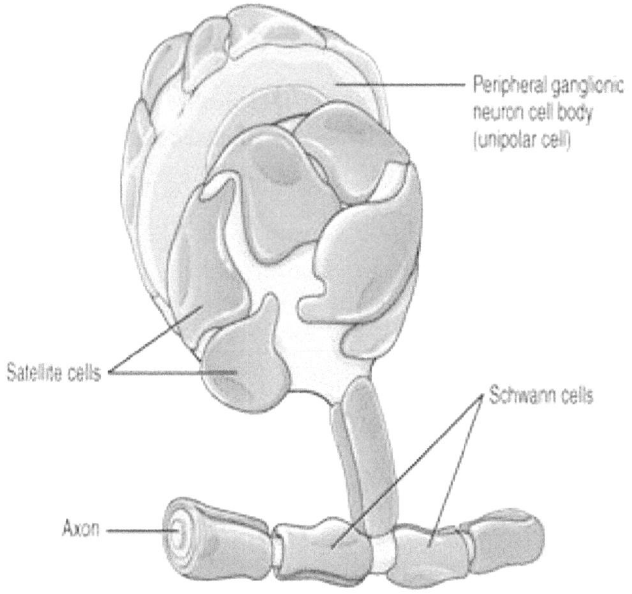

In the peripheral nervous system, which connects your brain and spinal cord to your limbs and organs, Schwann cells play a vital role. They form a protective covering over nerve fibers, aiding in rapid signal transmission. Some Schwann cells also assist in repairing damaged nerves, crucial for recovery from injuries.

OLIGODENDROCYTES: THE CENTRAL NERVOUS SYSTEM'S SUPPORT

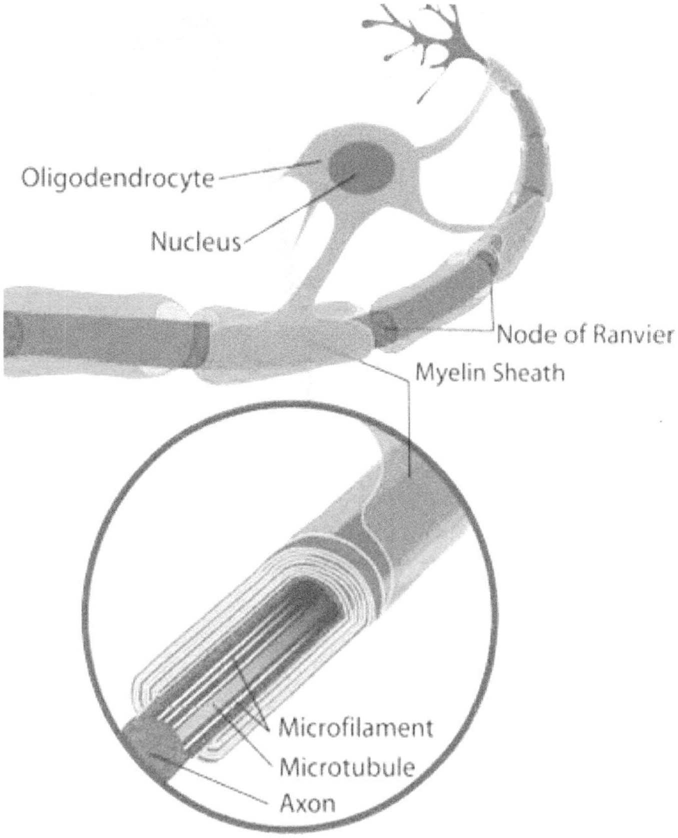

Oligodendrocytes, found in the central nervous system, perform a similar function to Schwann cells but with a broader reach, as a single oligodendrocyte can insulate up to 50 nerve fibers. This insulation is essential for preventing signal loss and ensuring speedy communication within the brain and spinal cord.

ASTROCYTES: THE DO-IT-ALL CELLS

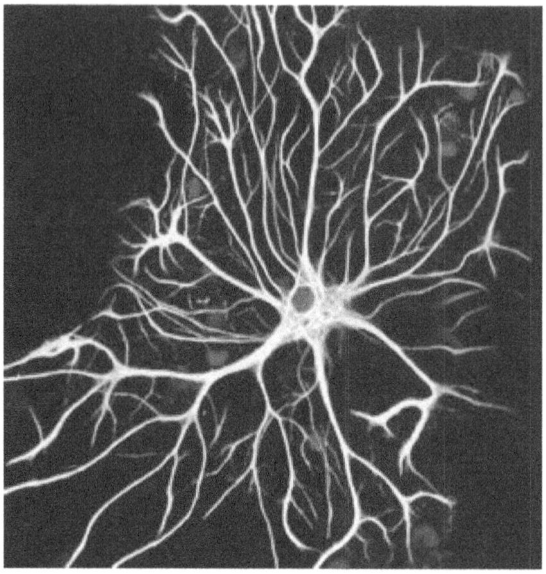

Astrocytes, an essential cell type in the central nervous system, play multifaceted roles crucial for brain function and health. They offer vital biochemical support to endothelial cells within the blood-brain barrier (BBB), ensuring that this critical boundary effectively regulates the passage of substances into the brain. Moreover, astrocytes are fundamental in providing nutrients to neurons, directly influencing neuronal health and functionality.

In response to brain injury, these cells are adept at repairing damage and forming scar tissue, which is key in the brain's healing process, albeit sometimes at the cost of inhibiting neuronal regeneration. A crucial aspect of their role involves maintaining ion balance in the brain, which is essential for normal brain function. This balancing act extends to helping regulate electrical impulses, ensuring that neuronal signaling remains effective and precise.

Astrocytes also contribute to vasomodulation, the process of controlling blood flow to different brain regions, which is vital for delivering nutrients and oxygen in response to neuronal activity. Beyond these functional roles, astrocytes also contribute significantly to the brain's physical structure, providing a scaffold that supports and organizes neurons and other brain cells. The multifunctionality of astrocytes underscores their importance in maintaining the brain's overall health and integrity.

MICROGLIAL CELLS: THE BRAIN'S IMMUNE WATCHERS

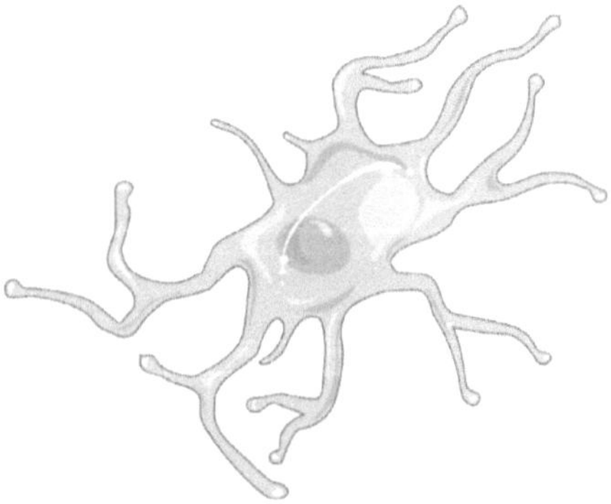

Microglial cells, making up about 10-15% of all brain cells, act as the immune system within the brain. They have the unique ability to transform based on the brain's needs – either monitoring their surroundings for potential threats or actively moving to address issues. Their adaptability is crucial for maintaining brain health.

EPENDYMAL CELLS: THE PRODUCERS OF CEREBROSPINAL FLUID

Ependymal cells have a specialized role in producing cerebrospinal fluid (CSF), a fluid that cushions and protects the brain and spinal cord. These cells line the spaces in the brain where CSF is found and use cilia to ensure its movement and distribution.

THE COLLECTIVE EFFORT FOR A HEALTHY NERVOUS SYSTEM

Together, these diverse cell types form a sophisticated network, ensuring the nervous system functions effectively. They provide structural and metabolic support, facilitate rapid signal transmission, engage in repair and defense mechanisms, and maintain the essential environment for neuronal function. It's a finely tuned system, with each cell type contributing to the overall health and efficiency of the brain and nervous system.

TASK 1: FILL IN THE BLANKS

1. Neurons are the primary cells in the brain and nervous system responsible for ________ and ________ signals.
2. The cerebral cortex contains between 10 to 20 _________ neurons, while the cerebellum has about 55 to 70 billion.
3. Schwann cells are found in the _________ nervous system and form a protective covering over nerve _________.
4. Oligodendrocytes are located in the _________ nervous system and can insulate up to ______ nerve fibres.
5. Microglial cells make up about 10-15% of all brain cells and act as the ________ system within the brain.
6. Ependymal cells produce _________ fluid, which cushions and protects the brain and spinal cord.
7. The role of Schwann cells and oligodendrocytes is crucial for preventing signal ______ and ensuring speedy _________ within the nervous system.
8. Microglial cells can transform to either monitor their surroundings or actively move to address _______ in the brain.
9. Cerebrospinal fluid is distributed in the brain by ependymal cells using _______.
10. The collective effort of neurons and various glial cells ensures the _________ system functions effectively.

TASK 2: LET'S TALK

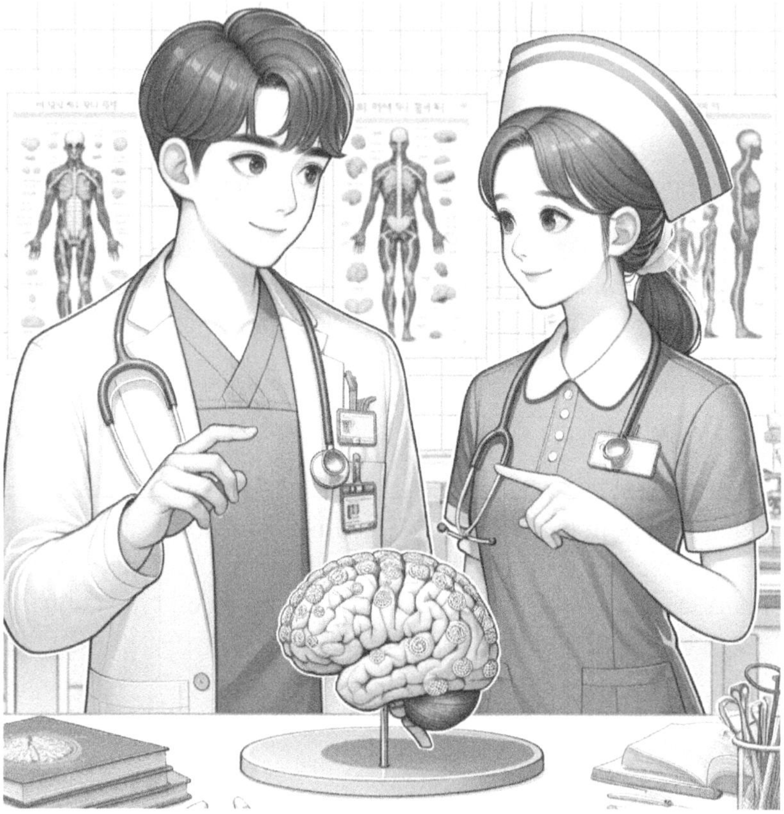

Alex: Hey Jamie, have you started studying for the neurology exam yet?

Jamie: Yeah, I've been trying to get my head around all these different cells in the nervous system. It's a lot to remember.

Alex: Tell me about it. I find the neurons fascinating, though. Did you know there are like 10-20 billion in the cerebral cortex alone?

Jamie: That's insane! And don't forget the cerebellum, with its 55-70 billion neurons. It's mind-blowing how many there are.

Alex: Exactly. And then there are the Schwann cells in the peripheral nervous system. They're like the protective layer for nerve fibers.

Jamie: Right, and they help with nerve repair, too. It's cool how they can wrap around the axons. But in the central nervous system, it's the oligodendrocytes that do the insulation work.

Alex: Yeah, a single oligodendrocyte can connect to up to 50 axons. That's efficiency for you. They're crucial for quick signal transmission.

Jamie: Don't forget about the microglial cells, the brain's own immune system. I read that they can change shape to react to different situations in the brain.

Alex: Oh, I remember reading that. They're like the brain's defenders. And then there are the ependymal cells that produce cerebrospinal fluid, right?

Jamie: Yep, the fluid that cushions our brain and spinal cord. Those cells use cilia to move the fluid around.

Alex: It's amazing how all these cells work together to make our nervous system function. Neurons for sending signals, glial cells for protection, support, and maintenance.

Jamie: Absolutely. It's like a well-coordinated team inside our body. Makes you appreciate how complex and wonderful the human body is.

Alex: Definitely. It's going to be interesting working with patients and applying this knowledge. Neurology is fascinating!

Jamie: Agreed. Let's ace this exam and get ready to put all this theory into practice!

TASK 3: DO YOU REMEMBER?

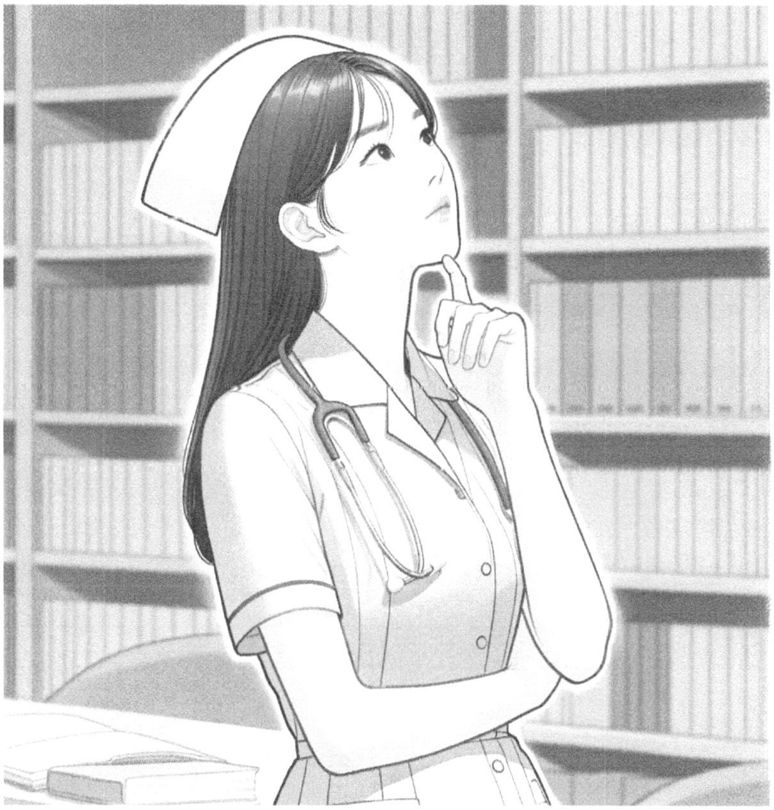

1. **What are the primary functions of neurons in the nervous system?**

____
____
____

2. **Approximately how many neurons are found in the cerebral cortex and the cerebellum?**

3. **What is the role of Schwann cells in the peripheral nervous system?**

4. **How do oligodendrocytes differ from Schwann cells in terms of their location and function?**

5. **What percentage of brain cells are made up of microglial cells, and what is their primary function?**

6. **What is the primary role of ependymal cells in the nervous system?**

7. **Why is the insulation of nerve fibers by Schwann cells and oligodendrocytes important for the nervous system?**

8. **How do microglial cells adapt to different situations in the brain?**

9. **What is the significance of cerebrospinal fluid, and how is it circulated in the brain?**

10. **Explain how the collective effort of neurons and various glial cells contributes to the functioning of the nervous system.**

TASK 4: LATIN AND GREEK TIME

1. **Neurons**
   - Derived from the Greek word "neuron" (νεῦρον), meaning nerve or sinew.
2. **Cerebral Cortex**
   - *Cerebral* comes from the Latin word "cerebrum," meaning brain.
   - *Cortex* comes from the Latin word "cortex," meaning bark or outer layer.
3. **Cerebellum**
   - Comes from the Latin word "cerebellum," meaning little brain.
4. **Sensory Neurons (Afferent Neurons)**
   - *Sensory* comes from the Latin word "sensōrius," meaning of or pertaining to the senses.
   - *Afferent* comes from the Latin word "afferens," meaning carrying towards.
5. **Motor Neurons (Efferent Neurons)**
   - *Motor* comes from the Latin word "motor," meaning mover.

- *Efferent* comes from the Latin word "efferens," meaning carrying away.

6. **Interneurons (Association Neurons)**

- *Inter-* comes from the Latin word "inter," meaning between.
- *Neurons* as above.
- *Association* comes from the Latin word "associare," meaning to unite or join.

7. **Pyramidal Cells**

- *Pyramidal* comes from the Latin word "pyramidalis," relating to a pyramid.

8. **Purkinje Cells**

- Named after Jan Evangelista Purkyně; the term itself does not have a Latin or Greek root.

9. **Unipolar Neurons**

- *Uni-* comes from the Latin word "unus," meaning one.
- *Polar* comes from the Greek word "polos" (πόλος), meaning axis or pole.

10. **Bipolar Neurons**

- *Bi-* comes from the Latin word "bis," meaning twice or double.
- *Polar* as above.

11. **Schwann Cells**

- Named after Theodor Schwann; the term itself does not have a Latin or Greek root.

12. **Oligodendrocytes**

- *Oligo-* comes from the Greek word "oligos" (ὀλίγος), meaning few or scanty.
- *Dendro-* comes from the Greek word "dendron" (δένδρον), meaning tree.
- *Cytes* comes from the Greek word "kytos" (κύτος), meaning container or cell.

13. **Microglial Cells**

- *Micro-* comes from the Greek word "mikros" (μικρός), meaning small.
- *Glial* comes from the Greek word "glia" (γλία), meaning glue.

14. **Ependymal Cells**

- Derived from the Greek word "ependyma" (ἐπένδυμα), meaning upper garment or tunic.

TASK 5: MAKE A CHOICE

1. What is the primary function of neurons?

A) Producing cerebrospinal fluid

B) Sending and receiving signals in the brain and nervous system

C) Forming a protective covering over nerve fibres

D) Acting as the immune system within the brain

2. What part of the brain contains between 10 to 20 billion neurons?

A) Cerebellum B) Cerebral cortex

C) Brainstem D) Medulla oblongata

3. Sensory neurons are responsible for:

A) Transmitting signals to muscles and glands

B) Converting external stimuli into internal electrical impulses

C) Connecting sensory and motor neurons

D) Motor control and coordination

4. Motor neurons transmit signals from:

A) The brain and spinal cord to the muscles and glands

B) Sensory organs to the brain

C) Neuron to neuron within the brain

D) The brain to the cerebellum

5. What do interneurons do?

A) Measure oxygen saturation levels

B) Control basic life-sustaining functions

C) Connect sensory and motor neurons

D) Produce cerebrospinal fluid

6. Where are Purkinje cells located?

A) Cerebral cortex B) Cerebellum

C) Peripheral nervous system D) Spinal cord

7. Schwann cells are found in the:

A) Central nervous system B) Peripheral nervous system C) Cerebellum D) Frontal lobe

8. Oligodendrocytes are similar to Schwann cells but are located in the:

A) Peripheral nervous system B) Central nervous system

C) Heart D) Lungs

9. Microglial cells function as what in the brain?

A) The immune system

B) Signal transmitters

C) Fluid producers

D) Oxygen carriers

10. Ependymal cells specialize in:

A) Transmitting nerve signals

B) Producing cerebrospinal fluid

C) Insulating nerve fibres

D) Repairing damaged nerves

Chapter 5: Grey Matter, White Matter, and Intelligence: Exploring sex Differences

The human brain is an intricate organ composed of various types of matter, each playing a unique role in cognitive function. Among these, grey and white matter stand out for their significant roles in determining intelligence (IQ).

GREY MATTER AND WHITE MATTER: FUNCTIONS AND COMPOSITION

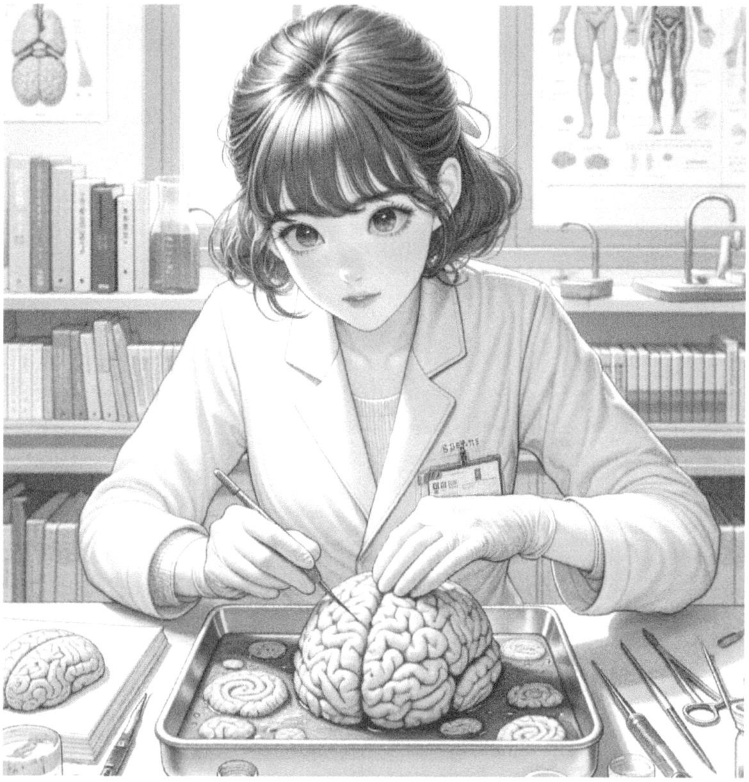

Grey Matter: Comprising neuron cell bodies, grey matter is fundamental in processing information in the brain. It is where most of the brain's synaptic connections occur.

White Matter: Consisting of axons, oligodendrocytes, and astrocytes, white matter is essential for communication within the brain. It forms the network through which different parts of the brain connect and communicate.

Research suggests that white matter is a crucial determinant of intelligence, influencing the speed and efficiency of neural connections.

THE QUESTION OF INTELLIGENCE: MEN VS. WOMEN

When comparing the average IQs of men and women, it's important to note that both genders have the same average IQ. However, the distribution and density of grey and white matter in their brains show notable differences:

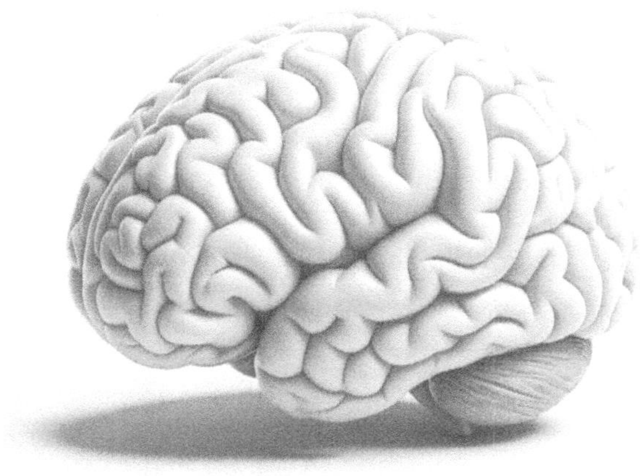

- **Male Brain**: On average, men's brains weigh 1,370 grams, with larger volumes or different neuronal densities in limbic and paralimbic regions.
- **Female Brain**: Women's brains, averaging 1,200 grams, have greater cortical grey matter volume relative to the size of the cerebrum. This includes larger volumes of regions associated with language functions, like Broca's area, and white matter involved in interhemispheric connectivity. Women also have a higher number of neurons per unit volume in areas like the planum temporale.

MALE AND FEMALE INSTINCTS AND COGNITIVE APPROACHES

- **Men**: Tend to adopt a more fact-based approach, focusing on defining and clarifying problems, and are good at focusing and eliminating irrelevant data.
- **Women**: Often take a more intuitive approach, perceiving events and people more deeply with greater memory capacity. They are inclined to define problems in broader terms and excel in holistic thinking.

SEX DIFFERENCES IN BRAIN DEVELOPMENT AND FUNCTION

- **Prefrontal Cortex**: In females, this region develops earlier than in males, leading to a larger prefrontal cortex in women, which aids in detail detection.

- **Amygdala**: Men have a larger amygdala, which is associated with threat detection.
- **Interhemispheric Connection**: This is 25% larger in females, which correlates with their ability to think in webs and contextualize ideas.

BRAIN HORMONES AND THEIR INFLUENCE

Oxytocin, known as the social attachment hormone, varies between genders:

- **In Females**: Increases with pleasant conversation and decreases when ignored.
- **In Males**: Must remain balanced, as excessive oxytocin can decrease testosterone levels and increase stress.

The differences in grey and white matter, along with variations in brain development and hormone levels, contribute to distinct cognitive styles in men and women. While men may excel in certain cognitive tasks, women may outperform in others, indicating a balance in intelligence across genders. Understanding these differences is crucial in appreciating the diverse strengths and capabilities inherent in the human brain.

TASK 1: FILL IN THE BLANKS

1. Grey matter in the brain is primarily made up of neuron _______ _______.
2. White matter consists of ________, oligodendrocytes, and _________.
3. _________ matter is important for determining intelligence, or IQ.
4. The average brain weight of males is ________ grams, while for females, it is ________ grams.
5. Females have a greater volume of grey matter in regions associated with _________ functions.
6. In the planum temporale, women have a higher number of _________ per unit volume than men.
7. Men typically use a more _______-based approach to problem-solving.
8. Women are known for their _________ thinking and greater memory capacity.
9. The _________ Cortex in females develops earlier and is larger than in males.
10. Oxytocin, a social attachment hormone, increases in females during _________ conversation.

TASK 2: LET'S TALK

Sarah: Hey David, have you read the latest research on brain differences between men and women? It's quite fascinating.

David: Oh, you mean the stuff about grey and white matter? Yeah, I skimmed through it. Grey matter is more about neuron cell bodies, right?

Sarah: Exactly. And white matter involves axons and glial cells like oligodendrocytes. It's interesting how these differences might relate to intelligence.

David: True. I was surprised to learn that white matter is linked with IQ. But what really caught my attention is that men and women have the same average IQ, despite these brain differences.

Sarah: I found that part about language functions in women intriguing. The study said women have greater cortical grey matter volume, especially in areas like Broca's area.

David: Yeah, and don't forget the part about the planum temporale. Women apparently have a higher number of neurons per unit volume there.

Sarah: It's all about the balance, I guess. Like how men tend to have a more fact-based approach, focusing on specific problems and getting rid of unnecessary data.

David: While women are more about intuitive and holistic thinking, right? They consider a wider array of factors before coming to a solution.

Sarah: Exactly! And there's also a difference in brain development. Like how the female prefrontal cortex develops earlier, which might explain why women take fewer risks in youth.

David: That's a good point. Also, the larger prefrontal cortex in women for detail detection contrasts with men's larger amygdala for threat detection.

Sarah: The hormone differences are interesting too. Oxytocin, the social attachment hormone, behaves differently in men and women.

David: Yes, it increases in women during pleasant conversations but needs to remain balanced in men. Too much can actually increase stress in males.

Sarah: All these insights are so valuable, especially in our field. Understanding these differences can really help in patient care and communication.

David: Absolutely, Sarah. It reminds us how unique each patient is and how these differences can influence their health and behaviour.

TASK 3: DO YOU REMEMBER?

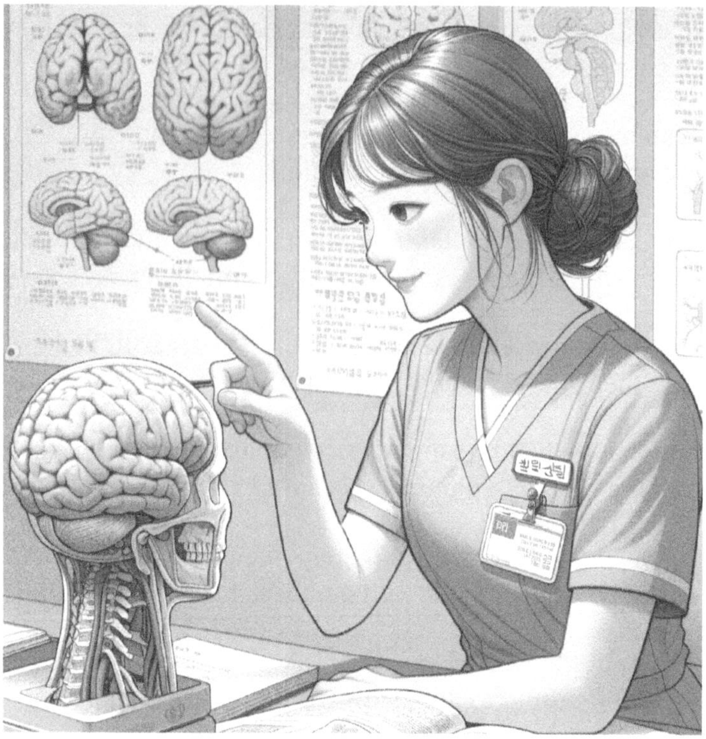

1. **What is primarily composed of neuron cell bodies: grey matter or white matter?**

2. **What does white matter mainly consist of?**

3. **How is white matter linked to intelligence or IQ?**

4. **What are the average brain weights for males and females, in grams?**

5. **In which brain regions do females typically have greater cortical grey matter volume?**

6. **Where do women have a higher number of neurons per unit volume compared to men?**

7. **What type of problem-solving approach is more common in men according to the article?**

8. **How do women generally approach problem-solving differently from men?**

9. **Which part of the brain develops earlier in females, and what risk-related behavior does this influence?**

10. **How does the hormone oxytocin behave differently in men and women?**

____

____

____

TASK 4: LATIN AND GREEK TIME

1. **Cognitive**
   - Comes from the Latin word "cognoscere," meaning to know or learn.
2. **Intelligence (IQ)**
   - *Intelligence* comes from the Latin word "intelligentia," meaning understanding.
   - *IQ* stands for "Intelligence Quotient," with "quotient" coming from the Latin word "quotiens," meaning how many times.
3. **Grey Matter**
   - *Grey* comes from the Old English word "grǣg," not directly from Latin or Greek.
   - *Matter* comes from the Latin word "materia," meaning substance or material.
4. **White Matter**
   - *White* comes from the Old English word "hwīt," not directly from Latin or Greek.
   - *Matter* as above.
5. **Neuron**
   - Derived from the Greek word "neuron" (νεῦρον), meaning nerve or sinew.
6. **Synaptic**
   - Comes from the Greek word "synapsis" (σύναψις), meaning conjunction or contact.
7. **Axons**
   - Derived from the Greek word "axon" (ἄξων), meaning axle or axis.
8. **Oligodendrocytes**
   - *Oligo-* comes from the Greek word "oligos" (ὀλίγος), meaning few or scanty.
   - *Dendro-* comes from the Greek word "dendron" (δένδρον), meaning tree.

- *Cytes* comes from the Greek word "kytos" (κύτος), meaning container or cell.

9. **Astrocytes**

- *Astro-* comes from the Greek word "astron" (ἄστρον), meaning star.
- *Cytes* as above.

10. **Cerebrum**

- Comes from the Latin word "cerebrum," meaning brain.

11. **Prefrontal Cortex**

- *Prefrontal* combines "pre-" (before, in front of) from Latin and "frontal" from "frontalis" in Latin, meaning of or belonging to the front.
- *Cortex* comes from the Latin word "cortex," meaning bark or outer layer.

12. **Amygdala**

- Derived from the Greek word "amygdale" (ἀμυγδαλή), meaning almond.

13. **Oxytocin**

- Comes from the Greek words "oxys" (ὀξύς), meaning quick, and "tokos" (τόκος), meaning childbirth.

Chapter 6: Physiology of the sexes

Understanding the physiological differences between men and women is crucial in various fields, including medicine, sports science, and nutrition. These distinctions, which are deeply rooted in our biology, manifest in various anatomical structures, hormonal levels, and even in psychological aspects. In this comprehensive analysis, we delve into the specifics of these differences, exploring their implications on health, risks, and benefits.

SEX DIFFERENCES IN SKULL ANATOMY

Forensic anthropology often utilizes skull features to determine sex. While there are exceptions, certain characteristics are typically more prevalent in male or female skulls:

1. **Forehead and Brow Ridge**: Male skulls usually have a sloping, less rounded forehead with a prominent supraorbital ridge, whereas female skulls tend to have a more rounded forehead with a smoother brow ridge.
2. **Eye Sockets**: Female skulls often feature round eye sockets with sharp upper margins, compared to the squarer orbits with blunter margins in male skulls.
3. **Jaw**: Males generally exhibit a square jawline with a vertical alignment from the outer edge of the jaw to the ear, while females typically have a more pointed jaw with a gentler slope towards the ear.

These differences are indicative rather than definitive, and a combination of features is usually analyzed to determine sex.

MUSCULAR AND FAT DISTRIBUTION DIFFERENCES

The disparity in muscle mass and fat distribution between the sexes has prfound implications on physical strength and health risks:

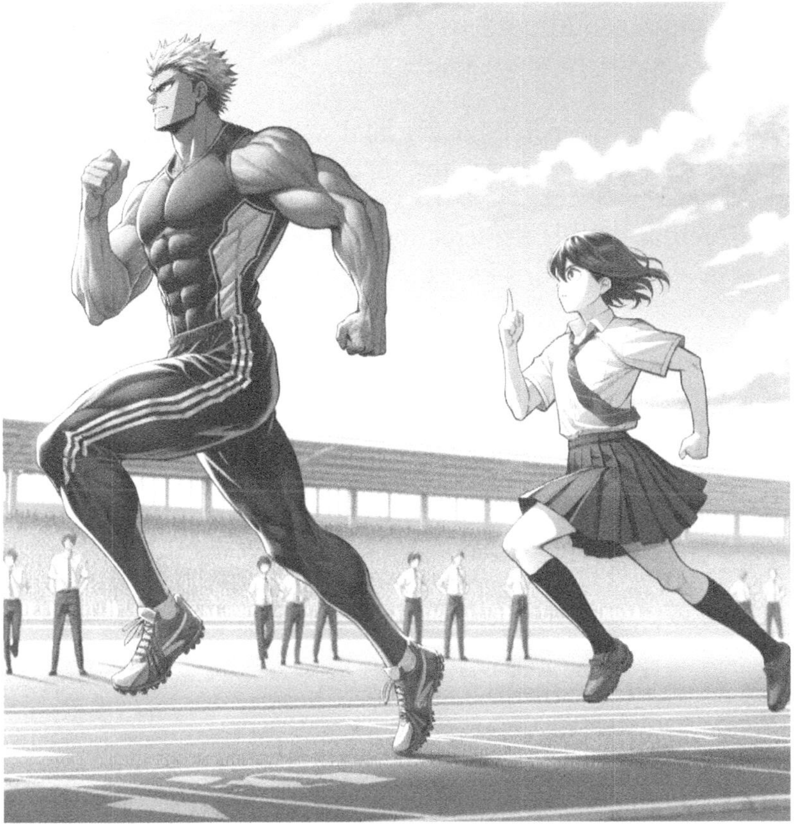

1. **Muscular Strength**: On average, females have about 40% less upper-body strength and 33% less lower-body strength compared to males, primarily due to differences in testosterone levels.

2. **Fat Distribution**: Women tend to have a higher percentage of body fat than men and store fat differently. Women's pattern of fat distribution, mostly around the hips and thighs, provides protection against metabolic diseases like type 2 diabetes and atherosclerosis.

HORMONAL INFLUENCES AND HEALTH IMPLICATIONS

Hormones play a critical role in the physiological differences between sexes:

1. **Estrogen and Bone Health**: Estrogen is linked with bone health and flexibility. Its fluctuation during the menstrual cycle correlates with the risk of knee and ankle injuries in women.

2. **Testosterone and Muscle Mass**: Higher testosterone in men contributes to increased muscle mass but also poses a risk for cardiovascular diseases if deficient.

ACL INJURIES AND WOMEN ATHLETES

Women athletes face a significantly higher risk of ACL injuries than men due to various physiological factors:

1. **Pelvic Width and Knee Alignment**: Women's wider pelvis changes the alignment and mechanics of the lower body, increasing stress on the ACL.
2. **Landing Mechanics**: Women typically land with a stiffer leg and do not bend as deeply as men during jumps, heightening the risk for knee injuries.
3. **Hormonal Fluctuations**: The fluctuation of estrogen during the menstrual cycle is potentially linked to increased laxity in women's knees, elevating injury risks.

THE Q-ANGLE

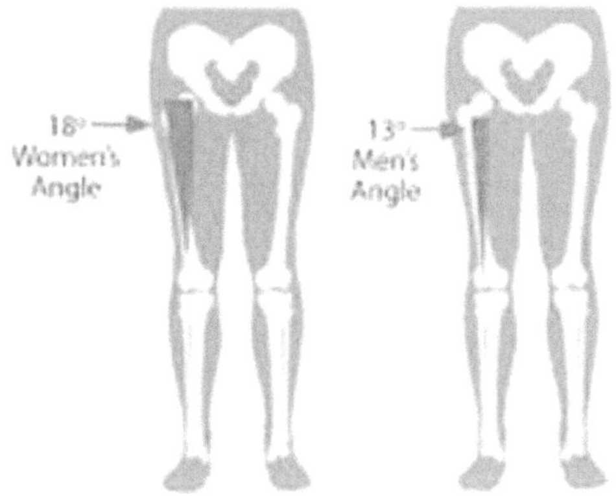

The quadriceps angle, or Q-Angle, varies significantly between men and women, affecting physical performance and injury risk:

1. **Increased Q-Angle in Women**: Leads to more pressure on the lower body, affecting stability and injury susceptibility.
2. **Decreased Q-Angle in Men**: Contributes to more torque and speed, influencing athletic performance.

HEALTH BENEFITS AND RISKS

The physiological differences between sexes not only influence physical capabilities but also impact health risks and benefits:

1. **Cardiovascular Health**: Estrogen in women has protective effects against heart disease, though this diminishes after menopause. Men's greater muscle mass, influenced by testosterone, is beneficial for strength but can increase the risk of cardiovascular diseases if testosterone levels drop significantly.
2. **Metabolic Disease Protection in Women**: Women's specific fat distribution pattern provides a degree of protection against metabolic diseases.

IMPLICATIONS FOR HEALTHCARE AND SPORTS

These physiological differences necessitate tailored approaches in healthcare, sports training, and injury prevention. Customized training programs can help mitigate injury risks, while understanding hormonal influences can guide more effective treatment strategies.

The physiological differences between men and women are vast and influential, extending beyond mere appearances to impact muscle strength, fat distribution, and disease risks. These distinctions necessitate personalized approaches in medicine, sports science, and nutrition to optimize health and well-being. By embracing and understanding these differences, we can better manage health risks and enhance physical and mental well-being for both sexes.

TASK 1: FILL IN THE BLANKS

1. Skull features used in forensic anthropology can indicate the _____ of an individual.
2. Male skulls typically have a _____ forehead with a prominent ________ ridge, while female skulls feature a more ________ forehead.
3. Female skulls often have round _____ sockets, compared to the squarer ones in male skulls.
4. Females generally have about _______% less upper-body strength than males, largely due to differences in _________ levels.
5. Women's pattern of fat distribution offers protection against diseases like _______ diabetes and _________.
6. Estrogen, a hormone linked to bone health, fluctuates during the menstrual cycle, affecting the risk of _______ injuries in women.
7. Higher levels of _________ in men contribute to increased muscle mass but can increase the risk of __________ diseases if deficient.
8. Women athletes have a higher risk of ______ injuries due to factors like pelvic width and landing mechanics.
9. The _________ angle, or Q-Angle, is different between men and women, affecting physical performance and injury risk.
10. In women, an increased Q-Angle leads to more pressure on the ______ body, while in men, a decreased Q-Angle creates more _______ and speed.
11. Estrogen provides protective effects against _______ disease in women, a benefit that diminishes after _________.
12. Understanding these physiological differences is crucial in fields like _________, sports science, and _________.

13. Tailored approaches in healthcare and sports training can help _______ injury risks and optimize ________ and mental well-being for both sexes.

TASK 2: LET'S TALK

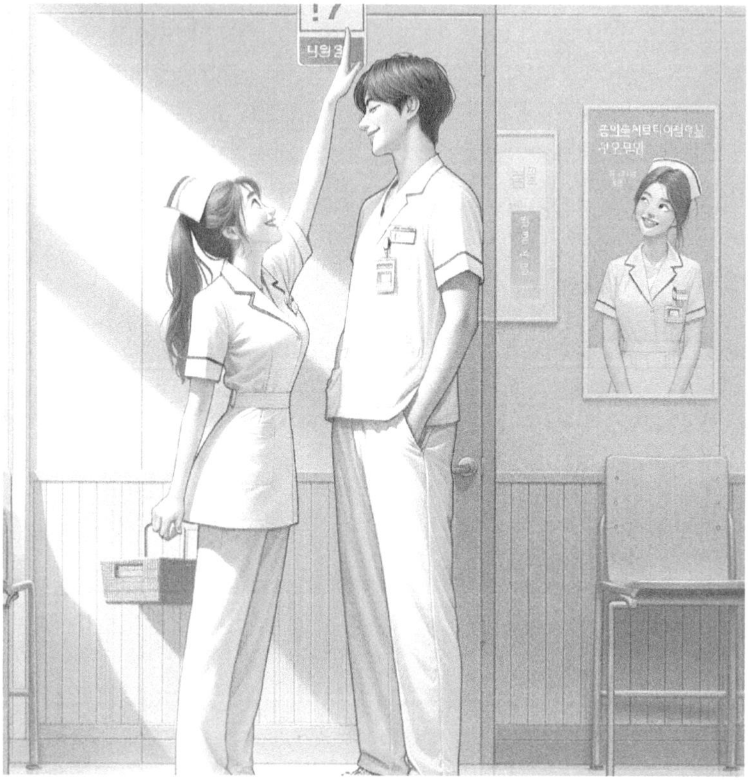

Hannah: Hey Carlos, have you noticed how our approaches to treatment sometimes have to change depending on whether the patient is male or female?

Carlos: Definitely, Hannah. The physiological differences can significantly influence how we administer care. Like how the risk of ACL injuries is higher in women, especially athletes. This means being more cautious with certain physical therapies and exercises.

Hannah: Right, that's because of their wider pelvis and different Q-angle, isn't it? It affects knee alignment and the stress on the ACL. We need to consider these anatomical differences in our rehabilitation plans.

Carlos: Exactly. And when it comes to cardiac issues, I read that symptoms of heart attacks can manifest differently in women compared to men. Women may experience more subtle symptoms, which means we have to be very attentive to their descriptions of discomfort.

Hannah: That's a great point. Also, considering hormonal fluctuations in women, especially how estrogen levels impact their susceptibility to certain injuries, is crucial. We need to factor these in when planning treatments, like when prescribing medications or suggesting lifestyle changes.

Carlos: And don't forget about muscle mass differences. Men generally have greater muscle mass due to higher testosterone levels, which can impact how we approach their physical therapies or strength training.

Hannah: Speaking of testosterone, its deficiency in men can lead to a range of health issues, including cardiovascular diseases. We have to be mindful of these risks when assessing male patients, especially older adults.

Carlos: True. In nutrition and weight management, the different fat distribution patterns between the sexes play a role too. Women tend to store more fat in the hips and thighs, while men store it around the abdomen, which is linked to higher cardiovascular risk.

Hannah: Absolutely, this means providing tailored dietary advice and exercise regimens. And for mental health, acknowledging these physiological differences helps in understanding how men and women might experience and express emotional issues differently.

Carlos: It all comes down to personalized care, doesn't it? Understanding these physiological differences helps us provide more effective and safer treatments.

Hannah: Yes, it's about seeing each patient as an individual and tailoring our care to their unique needs. It's fascinating how much there is to consider.

TASK 3: DO YOU REMEMBER?

1. **What physiological difference increases the risk of ACL injuries in women?**

____

____

____

2. **How does the Q-angle difference affect knee alignment in women?**

____

____

____

3. **Why might women experience heart attack symptoms differently from men?**

____

____

____

4. **How do hormonal fluctuations, particularly estrogen levels, influence women's susceptibility to certain injuries?**

5. **In what way does muscle mass, influenced by testosterone, differ between men and women?**

6. **What health issues can testosterone deficiency in men lead to?**

7. **How do fat distribution patterns differ between men and women, and what health risks are associated with these patterns?**

8. **Why is tailored dietary advice important considering the differences in fat distribution between sexes?**

9. **How can understanding physiological differences between sexes improve mental health treatment?**

10. **What does personalized care in nursing entail with respect to sex differences?**

11. **Why is it important for treatments to be gender-sensitive?**

12. **How can nurses adjust rehabilitation plans based on a patient's sex?**

13. **What considerations should be taken into account when prescribing medications to women?**

14. **What factors should be considered in physical therapies or strength training for men?**

15. **How do differences in heart attack symptoms between sexes impact nursing assessments?**

TASK 4: LATIN AND GREEK TIME

1. **Physiological**

    - Derived from the Greek words "physis" (φύσις), meaning nature, and "logia" (λογία), meaning study of.

2. **Anatomy**

    - Comes from the Greek word "anatomia" (ἀνατομία), composed of "ana" (ἀνά), meaning up, and "temnein" (τέμνειν), meaning to cut.

3. **Forensic**

    - Derived from the Latin word "forensis," meaning public or belonging to the forum.

4. **Anthropology**

    - Comes from the Greek words "anthropos" (ἄνθρωπος), meaning human, and "logia" (λογία), meaning study of.

5. **Estrogen**

    - Derived from the Greek words "oistros" (οἶστρος), meaning gadfly or frenzy, and "gen" (γένος), meaning producing.

6. **Testosterone**

    - *Testo-* is from the Latin word "testis," meaning witness or testicle.
    - *-sterone* is from the Greek word "ster" (στήρ), meaning solid, and the suffix "-one," indicating a ketone.

7. **Pelvic**

    - Comes from the Latin word "pelvis," meaning basin.

8. **Hormonal**

    - Derived from the Greek word "hormon" (ὁρμών), meaning setting in motion.

9. **Menstrual**

    - Comes from the Latin word "mensis," meaning month.

10. **Cardiovascular**

    - *Cardio-* comes from the Greek word "kardia" (καρδιά), meaning heart.

- *-vascular* comes from the Latin word "vasculum," meaning small vessel.

11. **Metabolic**

- Derived from the Greek word "metabole" (μεταβολή), meaning change.

12. **Quadriceps**

- *Quadri-* comes from the Latin word "quattuor," meaning four.
- *-ceps* comes from the Latin word "caput," meaning head.

13. **Healthcare**

- *Health* comes from the Old English word "hǣlth," not directly from Latin or Greek.
- *Care* comes from the Old English word "caru," meaning sorrow or anxiety, not directly from Latin or Greek.

14. **Nutrition**

- Derived from thc Latin word "nutrire," meaning to feed or nourish.

15. **Sports**

- Comes from the Old French word "desport," meaning leisure, not directly from Latin or Greek.

TASK 5: MAKE A CHOICE

1. What does forensic anthropology often use to determine sex?

A) DNA testing B) Blood tests

C) Skull features D) Height measurements

2. A characteristic typically more prevalent in male skulls is:

A) A more rounded forehead

B) Round eye sockets

C) A prominent supraorbital ridge

D) A pointed jaw with a gentler slope

3. Women tend to have a higher percentage of body fat compared to men, which is primarily stored:

A) In the abdominal region

B) Around the hips and thighs

C) In the upper body

D) Evenly distributed throughout the body

4. Estrogen is linked with:

A) Muscle mass development

B) Bone health and flexibility

C) Increased metabolic rate

D) Higher testosterone levels

5. Higher testosterone levels in men contribute to:

A) Decreased muscle mass

B) Improved cardiovascular health

C) Increased muscle mass

D) Lower risk of cardiovascular diseases

6. Women athletes have a higher risk of ACL injuries due to:

A) Lower estrogen levels

B) Pelvic width and knee alignment

C) Smaller muscle mass

D) Higher body fat percentage

7. The Q-Angle is significant because it:

A) Determines intellectual ability

B) Affects physical performance and injury risk

C) Measures body fat distribution

D) Indicates hormonal balance

8. After menopause, women's protection against heart disease:

A) Increases significantly B) Remains unchanged

C) Diminishes D) Depends on physical activity

9. Men's greater muscle mass can increase the risk of cardiovascular diseases if:

A) Muscle mass decreases significantly

B) Testosterone levels increase

C) Testosterone levels drop significantly

D) Estrogen levels increase

10. In healthcare and sports science, understanding physiological differences between sexes is crucial for:

A) Designing gender-neutral treatment plans

B) Tailoring approaches in treatment and training

C) Focusing solely on genetic factors

D) Implementing identical nutritional plans for both sexes

Chapter 7: Effective Management of Wounds and Understanding Venomous Bites

In the world of healthcare, particularly in emergency medicine, understanding different types of wounds and the appropriate first aid responses is crucial. Additionally, a comprehensive knowledge of how to handle venomous bites, particularly snakebites, is essential for both healthcare professionals and the general public.

DECIPHERING WOUND TYPES

INCISION WOUND:

Characterized by a clean, straight cut often inflicted by sharp objects like knives. Such wounds may appear deceptively benign but can be deep, affecting underlying tissues.

LACERATION WOUND:

These are irregular, jagged wounds typically caused by accidents involving blunt trauma. They are more prone to infection and require careful cleaning and closure.

ABRASION:

A surface wound that occurs when skin is scraped off, usually not very deep but painful and susceptible to infection.

PUNCTURE WOUND:

Caused by an object puncturing the skin, such as a nail. These wounds might look small but can be deep and prone to internal infections.

PENETRATION WOUND:

Occurs when an object enters the body, creating an open channel that can reach internal organs, posing a high risk of serious infection and internal damage.

CONTUSION:

Commonly known as a bruise, it results from blunt force causing blood vessels to rupture under the skin.

HEMATOMA:

A collection of blood outside the blood vessels, often appearing as a lump or bruise. It results from trauma or injury to the blood vessels.

FIRST AID ESSENTIALS FOR WOUND MANAGEMENT

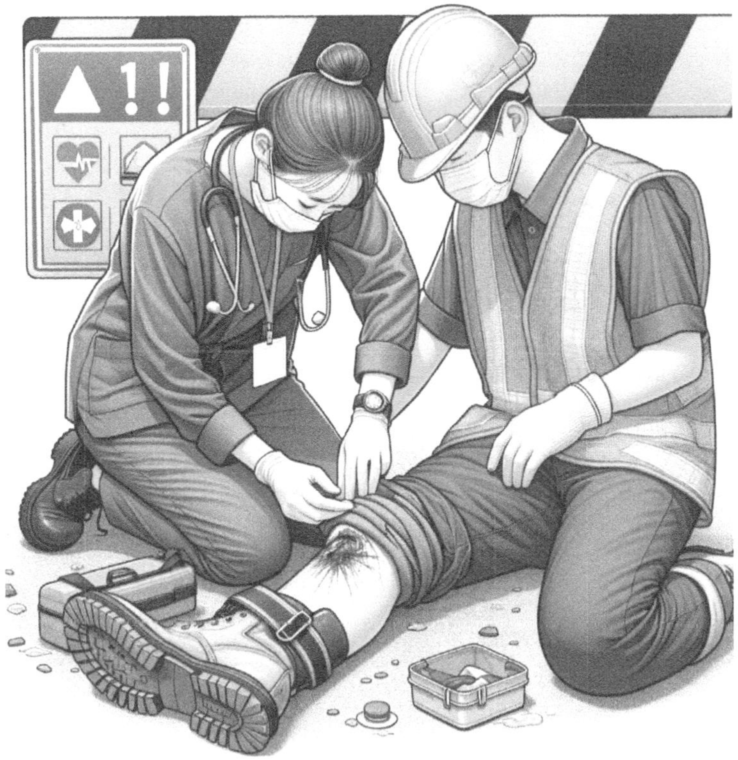

ELEVATION:

Raising the injured area above heart level reduces bleeding and swelling.

DIRECT PRESSURE:

Applying pressure directly to the wound site helps control bleeding. This is often the first and most effective step in bleeding control.

COLD PACK:

Used for bruises and contusions, cold packs reduce swelling and bleeding by constricting blood vessels.

PRESSURE BANDAGE:

Ideal for persistent bleeding, a pressure bandage applies steady pressure to stem blood flow.

MANAGING SNAKEBITES

IMMEDIATE ACTION:

Keep the bitten area immobilized and lower than the heart to reduce venom spread. Remove constricting items like rings or bracelets.

FIRST AID MYTHS:

Avoid cutting the wound or attempting to suck out venom. Ice application is also discouraged.

UNDERSTANDING ANTIBIOTICS AND RABIES

Antibiotics are crucial in preventing or treating infections that may arise from wounds. These substances, which can be natural or synthetic, work by inhibiting or destroying bacteria.

Rabies is a severe viral infection transmitted through animal bites. Early symptoms like fever and headache progress to severe neurological symptoms. Immediate medical attention and vaccination are critical.

THE DANGER OF VENOMS

Venoms, particularly from snakes like the Mamushi, pose a significant health risk. They contain toxins that can affect the nervous system (neurotoxins) or blood (hemotoxins). Antivenom is the primary treatment, and in some cases, an incision might be made to remove the venom from a bite site.

Understanding the types of wounds and their appropriate first aid responses, alongside knowledge of venomous bites, is essential in emergency healthcare. This knowledge not only aids in providing immediate care but also in preventing complications and ensuring the best possible outcomes for patients.

TASK 1: FILL IN THE BLANKS

1. An **Incision Wound** is typically caused by a _____ object and results in a clean, ______ cut.
2. A **Laceration Wound** is characterized by its ______, ______ edges.
3. **Abrasion** wounds are superficial, affecting primarily the _______ layer of the skin.
4. A **Puncture Wound** is caused by a ______ object and can be deceptively ______ despite its small appearance.
5. **Penetration Wound** occurs when an object ______ the body, potentially reaching ______ organs.
6. A **Contusion** is commonly known as a _______, caused by blunt force.
7. **Hematoma** is a collection of ______ outside of blood vessels, often appearing as a lump or ______.

8. To control bleeding, the injured area should be ______ above the heart level.

9. Applying ______ pressure is a critical first step in managing bleeding.

10. In the case of snakebite, it is important to keep the bitten area ______ and avoid ______ out the venom.

11. **Antibiotics** are used to treat or prevent infections by ______ or killing bacteria.

12. **Rabies** is a viral disease transmitted through the bite of a ______ animal.

13. **Venom** from creatures like the Mamushi snake can contain _______ affecting the nervous system or blood.

TASK 2: LET'S TALK

Liam: Emma, we've got a patient coming in with a deep cut on his arm. Looks like an incision wound.

Emma: Got it, Liam. It's probably from something sharp. We'll need to clean it and check for any underlying tissue damage. Incisions can be deeper than they appear.

Liam: Agreed. Oh, and did you hear about the construction worker who came in earlier with a nail in his foot?

Emma: Yes, I did. Classic puncture wound, right? Those can be tricky because of the risk of infection deep inside.

Liam: Exactly. We had to be careful with the cleaning and antibiotics. There's also a kid in the waiting room who fell off his bike. He's got a nasty abrasion on his knee.

Emma: Poor thing. Abrasions can be so painful, even if they're mostly superficial. We'll need to clean it thoroughly to prevent infection.

Liam: Speaking of infections, have you updated your rabies vaccination? We've had a few animal bite cases this month.

Emma: Yes, I'm up to date with my shots. Rabies is no joke. The initial flu-like symptoms can escalate quickly into something much more serious.

Liam: True. By the way, did you handle the snakebite case last week?

Emma: I did. We had to keep the patient's limb immobilized and lower than the heart. Luckily, we got the antivenom in time. Remember, no cutting or sucking the venom.

Liam: Good call. Managing venomous bites can be intense. Did you know some venoms act as neurotoxins, affecting the nervous system?

Emma: Yeah, and others are hemotoxins, affecting the blood. Every case is unique. It's why I love working in the ER. You never know what's going to come through that door.

Liam: Exactly. It keeps us on our toes and always learning. Alright, let's get ready for the next patient.

TASK 3: DO YOU REMEMBER?

1. **What is the main difference between an incision wound and a laceration wound in terms of how they look?**

____

____

____

2. **Why is it important to clean a laceration wound carefully?**

____

____

____

3. **Describe what an abrasion wound is and what the main concern is when treating it.**

____

____

____

4. **Explain what a puncture wound is and why it might be more serious than it appears.**

____

____

____

5. **What does a penetration wound involve, and why are they considered high risk?**

____

____

____

6. **What is a contusion, and how is it commonly caused?**

7. **Define a hematoma and explain how it differs from a simple bruise.**

8. **In terms of first aid, what is the purpose of applying direct pressure to a bleeding wound?**

9. **What are the initial steps that should be taken if someone is bitten by a snake?**

10. **Why is it important for everyone, not just healthcare professionals, to understand the basics of different wound types and their first aid treatment?**

TASK 4: LATIN AND GREEK TIME

1. **Incision**

    - Comes from the Latin word "incisio," meaning a cutting into.

2. **Laceration**

- Derived from the Latin word "lacerare," meaning to tear or mangle.

3. **Abrasion**
   - Comes from the Latin word "abrasio," meaning a scraping.
4. **Puncture**
   - Derived from the Latin word "punctura," meaning a pricking.
5. **Penetration**
   - Comes from the Latin word "penetrare," meaning to put or get into.
6. **Contusion**
   - Derived from the Latin word "contusio," meaning a bruising.
7. **Hematoma**
   - *Hema-* comes from the Greek word "haima" (αἷμα), meaning blood.
   - *-toma* comes from the Greek word "toma" (τόμα), meaning a slice or piece.
8. **Elevation**
   - Comes from the Latin word "elevatio," meaning a lifting up.
9. **Antibiotics**
   - *Anti-* comes from the Greek word "anti" (ἀντί), meaning against.
   - *Bio-* comes from the Greek word "bios" (βίος), meaning life.
   - *-tics* is from the Greek word "tikos" (τικός), relating to making or producing.
10. **Rabies**
    - Comes from the Latin word "rabies," meaning madness or rage.
11. **Venom**
    - Derived from the Latin word "venenum," meaning poison.
12. **Neurotoxins**
    - *Neuro-* comes from the Greek word "neuron" (νεῦρον), meaning nerve.
    - *-toxins* comes from the Greek word "toxikon" (τοξικόν), meaning poison for arrows.

13. **Hemotoxins**

- *Hemo-* as in hematoma.
- *-toxins* as in neurotoxins.

14. **Antivenom**

- *Anti-* as in antibiotics.
- *Venom* as above.

15. **Mamushi**

- A specific type of snake, not derived from Latin or Greek.

TASK 5: MAKE A CHOICE

1. What is an incision wound typically caused by?

A) Blunt trauma B) Sharp objects like knives

C) Scraping against a rough surface D) Animal bites

2. What characterizes a laceration wound?

A) A clean, straight cut B) A jagged, irregular wound

C) A small, deep hole D) Surface-level scraping

3. An abrasion is a wound that:

A) Occurs when skin is scraped off

B) Involves puncturing of the skin

C) Is a deep cut into the skin

D) Results from a blunt force

4. A puncture wound is caused by:

A) An object puncturing the skin

B) A sharp cut to the skin

C) Blunt force trauma

D) Scratching the skin surface

5. A penetration wound is characterized by:

A) An object entering the body and reaching internal organs

B) A superficial injury to the skin

C) A closed injury with ruptured blood vessels

D) Surface-level scraping

6. A contusion is commonly known as:

A) A scrape B) A bruise C) A cut D) A puncture

7. What is a hematoma?

A) A type of abrasion

B) A collection of blood outside the blood vessels

C) A small puncture wound

D) A cut with jagged edges

8. In first aid, elevation of the injured area is used to:

A) Reduce bleeding and swelling

B) Increase blood flow to the area

C) Cool the wound

D) Prevent infection

9. What role do hormones play in physiological differences between sexes?

A) They have no significant role

B) They influence muscle mass and fat distribution

C) They determine skin type

D) They only affect emotional responses

10. Managing snakebites involves:

A) Keeping the bitten area immobile and lower than the heart

B) Applying ice to the wound

C) Cutting the wound to release venom

D) Sucking out the venom

Chapter 8: The Fundamentals of Immunology

Immunology, the study of the body's self-defense system, is a fascinating and complex field that plays a crucial role in maintaining health. It hinges on the immune system's ability to distinguish between self and non-self entities, a vital process for protecting the body from foreign invaders while avoiding damage to its own tissues. A malfunction in this system can lead to autoimmune diseases, where the body mistakenly attacks itself.

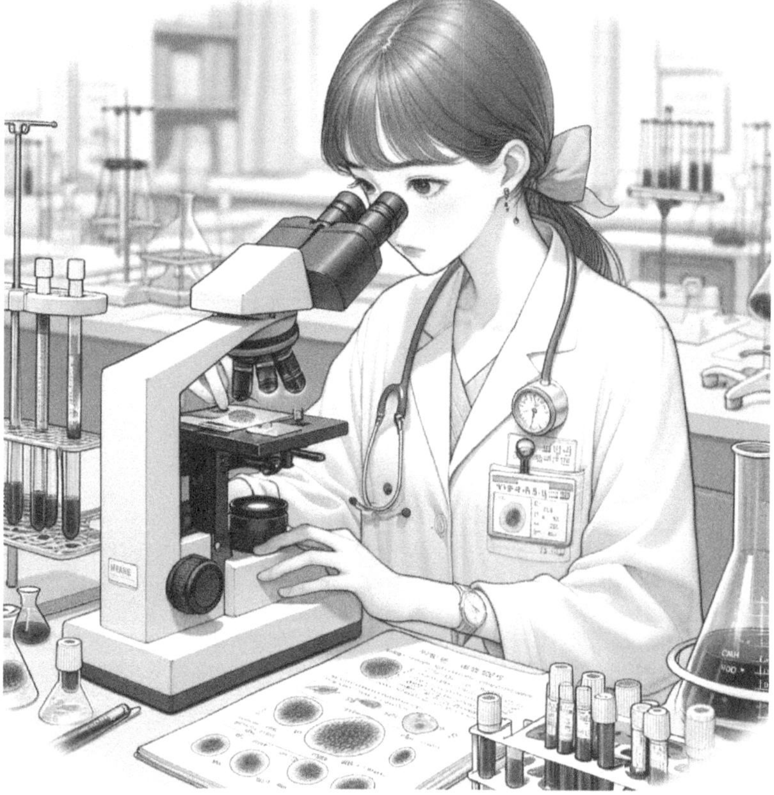

UNDERSTANDING INNATE VS. ADAPTIVE IMMUNITY

INNATE IMMUNITY:

Innate immunity is the body's first line of defense, offering nonspecific protection against pathogens. It is immediate and involves mechanisms like physical barriers (skin), chemicals in the blood, and immune cells that target foreign cells. The innate response is triggered by the antigen's chemical properties.

ADAPTIVE IMMUNITY:

Adaptive immunity is a specific response to an antigen. Unlike innate immunity, it is more complex and involves the processing and recognition of antigens. Once an antigen is identified, the adaptive system creates cells specialized in attacking that particular antigen. This system also retains a "memory" of the antigen, making future responses more efficient.

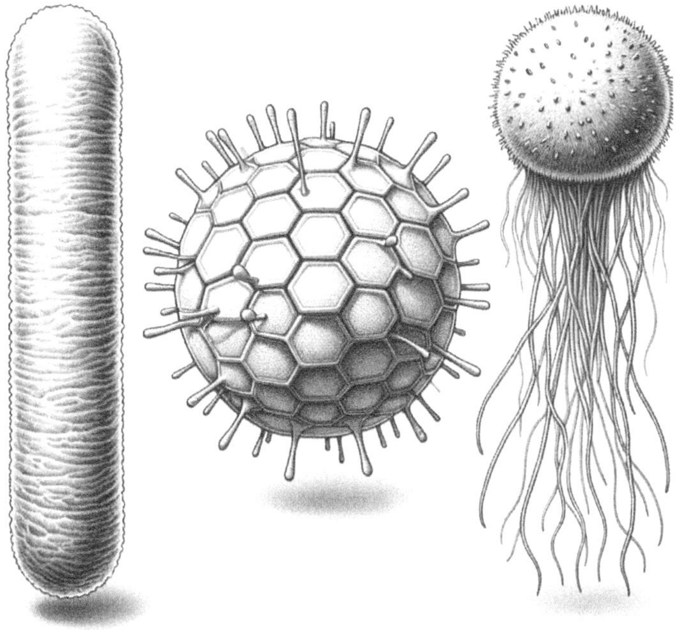

THE ROLE OF CYTOKINES AND CYTOTOXINS

CYTOKINES:

These are small proteins crucial in cell signaling, especially within the immune system. Produced by a range of cells, including macrophages and lymphocytes, cytokines are pivotal in health and disease, playing roles in immune responses, inflammation, and various diseases.

CYTOTOXINS:

Cytotoxins are substances toxic to cells, utilized by T cells for two main functions: cell lysis (disrupting the cell membrane) and apoptosis (cell self-destruction). They are essential in combating cancer cells, bacteria, fungi, and virus-infected cells.

BASIC IMMUNE CELLS AND THEIR FUNCTIONS

ANTIGENS AND ANTIBODIES:

An antigen is a molecule that triggers an immune response. Antibodies, or immunoglobulins, are Y-shaped proteins that neutralize pathogens by recognizing specific antigens. Each antibody is tailored to a specific antigen, allowing precise identification and response.

PRESENTATION OF ANTIGENS:

- **Class I MHC Molecules**: These are displayed by all nucleated cells and present endogenously generated antigens.

- **Class II MHC Molecules**: These present extracellular antigens and are found on professional antigen-presenting cells (APCs) like dendritic cells and macrophages.

MYELOID AND LYMPHOID CELLS: KEY PLAYERS IN IMMUNITY

DENDRITIC CELLS:

Act as messengers between innate and adaptive immunity. They process antigens and present them to T cells.

BASOPHILS AND EOSINOPHILS:

Basophils play a role in allergic reactions and inflammation, while eosinophils combat multicellular parasites and certain infections.

NEUTROPHILS AND MACROPHAGES:

Neutrophils are abundant granulocytes responding to inflammation. Macrophages rid the body of debris and present antigens.

MAST CELLS AND MEGAKARYOCYTES:

Mast cells are involved in wound healing and defense against pathogens. Megakaryocytes produce platelets for blood clotting.

NATURAL KILLER CELLS AND T-CELLS:

NK cells recognize and destroy stressed cells without needing antibodies or MHC. T-cells, differentiated in the thymus, are critical for identifying and destroying infected or foreign cells.

DELVING INTO T-CELL SUBTYPES

T-cells are diverse, with each subtype playing a unique role in immune defense and regulation. They include:

- **Helper CD4+ T Cells**: Assist other immune cells, produce cytokines, and are involved in autoimmune diseases.

- **Cytotoxic CD8+ T Cells**: Destroy virus-infected and tumor cells.

- **Regulatory CD4+ T Cells**: Maintain immunological tolerance.

- **Memory T Cells**: Remember antigens and can rapidly respond to previously encountered pathogens.

ADVANCED ANTIGEN-PRESENTING CELLS

Antigen-presenting cells can be professional (expressing MHC class II molecules) or non-professional (expressing MHC class I). These include dendritic cells, macrophages, and B cells.

In conclusion, the study of immunology reveals a sophisticated and dynamic system that protects our bodies from countless threats. Understanding its components and mechanisms is essential for developing treatments for various diseases and for advancing our knowledge of human health and disease.

TASK 1: FILL IN THE BLANKS

1. Immunology is the study of the body's ______-defense system.
2. The immune system must differentiate between ______ (non-self) and ______ (self) cells.
3. A condition where the immune system attacks the body is known as "_________ Disease."
4. ______ immunity is the body's first line of defense and responds to antigens immediately.
5. ______ immunity involves a specific response and has a "memory" component for future responses.
6. ______ are small proteins important in cell signaling and the immune system.
7. T cells use ______ to cause cell lysis and apoptosis.
8. Antigens are "targeted" by ______, also known as immunoglobulins.
9. Class I MHC molecules present _______ generated antigens.
10. Dendritic cells act as _______ between the innate and adaptive immune systems.
11. Basophils play a significant role in ______ reactions and inflammation.
12. ______ cells are a type of cytotoxic lymphocyte critical to the innate immune system.
13. Helper CD4+ T cells assist other lymphocytes and produce _______.

TASK 2: LET'S TALK

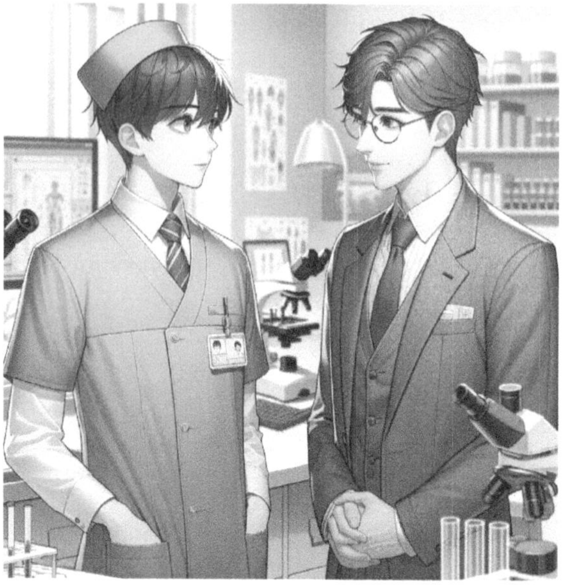

Jordan: Good morning, Dr. Simmons. I have a few questions about the immunology article we read for class.

Dr. Simmons: Of course, Jordan. What would you like to know?

Jordan: First, could you explain more about the difference between innate and adaptive immunity?

Dr. Simmons: Certainly. Innate immunity is your body's initial response to pathogens. It's non-specific and responds immediately to threats using physical barriers like skin and chemicals in the blood. Adaptive immunity, on the other hand, is more complex and specific. It develops after exposure to a specific pathogen and creates a memory for faster response in future encounters.

Jordan: That makes sense. And what about autoimmune diseases? What exactly happens there?

Dr. Simmons: In autoimmune diseases, the body's immune system mistakenly identifies its own cells as foreign and attacks them. It's a failure in the immune system's ability to distinguish between self and non-self.

Jordan: I see. Also, the article mentioned cytokines. What role do they play?

Dr. Simmons: Cytokines are crucial in cell signaling within the immune system. They are produced by various immune cells and are involved in responses to infection, inflammation, and other immune challenges.

Jordan: And cytotoxins, they are used by T cells, right?

Dr. Simmons: Exactly. T cells use cytotoxins for two main purposes: cell lysis, where they cause the infected cell's membrane to rupture, and apoptosis, which is the programmed cell death. This is important in controlling infections and eliminating cancer cells.

Jordan: What about the antigens and antibodies? How do they work together?

Dr. Simmons: Antigens are substances that trigger an immune response. Antibodies are proteins produced by the immune system that specifically target and neutralize these antigens. Each antibody is designed to match a specific antigen, like a lock and key.

Jordan: Got it. And dendritic cells, they're a link between the innate and adaptive immune systems?

Dr. Simmons: Precisely. Dendritic cells process antigens and present them to T cells, effectively communicating between the innate and adaptive systems.

Jordan: That's fascinating. And basophils, are they the ones involved in allergic reactions?

Dr. Simmons: Yes, basophils release chemicals like histamine during allergic reactions and inflammation. They're a small but important part of the immune response.

Jordan: Thank you, Dr. Simmons. This really clarifies a lot for me.

Dr. Simmons: You're welcome, Jordan. Always happy to discuss and clarify. Understanding these concepts is fundamental in nursing.

TASK 3: DO YOU UNDERSTAND?

1. **What is the primary focus of study in immunology?**

____
____
____

2. **What critical function does the immune system perform in distinguishing cell types?**

____
____
____

3. **What is an autoimmune disease, and how does it occur?**

____
____
____

4. **Describe the difference between innate immunity and adaptive immunity.**

5. **What are cytokines, and what role do they play in the immune system?**

6. **How do T cells use cytotoxins, and for what purposes?**

7. **What is the function of antigens in the immune system?**

8. **How do antibodies work in relation to antigens?**

9. **What is the role of dendritic cells in the immune system?**

10. **How are basophils involved in allergic reactions?**

TASK 4: LATIN AND GREEK TIME

1. **Immunology**

   - Derived from the Latin word "immunis" (free, exempt) and the Greek word "logia" (λογία), meaning the study of.

2. **Innate**

   - Comes from the Latin word "innatus," meaning inborn or natural.

3. **Adaptive**

   - Derived from the Latin word "adaptare," meaning to adjust or fit.

4. **Cytokines**

   - *Cyto-* comes from the Greek word "kytos" (κύτος), meaning cell.
   - *-kines* comes from the Greek word "kinesis" (κίνησις), meaning movement.

5. **Cytotoxins**

   - *Cyto-* as above.
   - *Toxins* comes from the Greek word "toxikon" (τοξικόν), meaning poison.

6. **Antigens**

   - *Anti-* comes from the Greek word "anti" (ἀντί), meaning against.
   - *-gens* comes from the Greek word "gennan" (γεννᾶν), meaning to produce.

7. **Antibodies** (Immunoglobulins)

   - *Anti-* as above.
   - *Bodies* comes from the Latin word "corpus," meaning body.
   - *Immunoglobulins* combine "immunis" from Latin and "globulus" (small sphere) from Latin.

8. **MHC (Major Histocompatibility Complex)**

- *Major* comes from the Latin word "major," meaning greater.
- *Histocompatibility* combines "histo-" from the Greek "histos" (ἱστός), meaning tissue, and "compatibility" from the Latin "compatibilis," meaning compatible.

9. **Dendritic**

- Derived from the Greek word "dendron" (δένδρον), meaning tree.

10. **Basophils**

- *Baso-* comes from the Greek word "basis" (βάσις), meaning base.
- *-phils* comes from the Greek word "philos" (φίλος), meaning loving or fond of.

11. **Eosinophils**

- *Eosin-* is from the Greek word "eos" (ἠώς), meaning dawn (referring to the color).
- *-phils* as above.

12. **Neutrophils**

- *Neutro-* comes from the Latin word "neuter," meaning neither.
- *-phils* as above.

13. **Macrophages**

- *Macro-* comes from the Greek word "makros" (μακρός), meaning large.
- *-phages* comes from the Greek word "phagein" (φαγεῖν), meaning to eat.

14. **Mast Cells**

- *Mast* comes from the Greek word "mastos" (μαστός), meaning breast, used here in the sense of a cell filled with granules.

15. **Megakaryocytes**

- *Mega-* comes from the Greek word "megas" (μέγας), meaning large.
- *Karyo-* comes from the Greek word "karyon" (κάρυον), meaning nut or kernel.
- *-cytes* comes from the Greek word "kytos" (κύτος), meaning cell.

16. **T-Cells**

- *T-* stands for thymus, where they mature, derived from the Greek word "thymos" (θυμός), meaning warty outgrowth or soul.

17. **B-Cells**

- *B-* stands for bursa of Fabricius in birds, where they were first discovered. "Bursa" is Latin for purse.

18. **Immunological Tolerance**

- *Immunological* as in immunology.
- *Tolerance* comes from the Latin word "tolerantia," meaning endurance.

TASK 5: MAKE A CHOICE

1. *Tolerance* comes from the Latin word "tolerantia," meaning endurance.

A) The body's digestive process

B) The body's self-defense system

C) The body's circulatory system

D) The body's reproductive system

2. What distinguishes innate immunity from adaptive immunity?

A) Innate immunity is a specific response to an antigen.

B) Innate immunity offers nonspecific protection against pathogens.

C) Innate immunity involves only chemical barriers.

D) Innate immunity retains a memory of antigens.

3. What characterizes adaptive immunity?

A) It provides immediate defense.

B) It creates cells specialized in attacking specific antigens.

C) It only involves physical barriers.

D) It does not have a memory system.

4. What is the role of cytokines in the immune system?

A) To act as physical barriers

B) To produce antibodies

C) To aid in cell signaling

D) To directly attack pathogens

5. Cytotoxins are used by T cells primarily for:

A) Creating memory cells

B) Cell lysis and apoptosis

C) Producing more T cells

D) Acting as physical barriers

6. What triggers an immune response in the body?

A) Antibodies B) Cytokines C) Antigens D) Platelets

7. What is the primary function of antibodies?

A) To warm the body B) To neutralize pathogens

C) To create antigens D) To act as messengers

8. What is the role of dendritic cells in immunity?

A) They produce antibodies

B) They act as messengers between innate and adaptive immunity

C) They destroy infected cells

D) They regulate body temperature

9. Basophils are mainly involved in:

A) Blood clotting

B) Allergic reactions and inflammation

C) Oxygen transport

D) Memory formation

10. The primary function of neutrophils is:

A) Responding to inflammation B) Healing wounds

C) Producing cytokines D) Neutralizing antigens

11. What is the role of natural killer (NK) cells?

A) To produce antibodies

B) To recognize and destroy stressed cells

C) To process antigens

D) To aid in digestion

12. Helper CD4+ T cells are involved in:

A) Blood clotting

B) Assisting other immune cells and producing cytokines

C) Directly attacking pathogens

D) Carrying oxygen

13. Cytotoxic CD8+ T cells primarily function to:

A) Destroy virus-infected and tumor cells

B) Produce antibodies

C) Act as physical barriers

D) Warm the body

14. What is the main function of regulatory CD4+ T cells?

A) To maintain immunological tolerance

B) To remember antigens

C) To produce platelets

D) To aid in digestion

15. Memory T cells are important because they:

A) Produce antibodies

B) Remember antigens for rapid response in the future

C) Act as the first line of defense

D) Are involved in allergic reactions

Chapter 9: The Pulmonary System

The pulmonary system, commonly referred to as the respiratory system, is an intricate and vital part of the human body. It is primarily responsible for the exchange of oxygen and carbon dioxide between the body and the environment, a process essential for life. This article explores the various components of the pulmonary system and their respective functions.

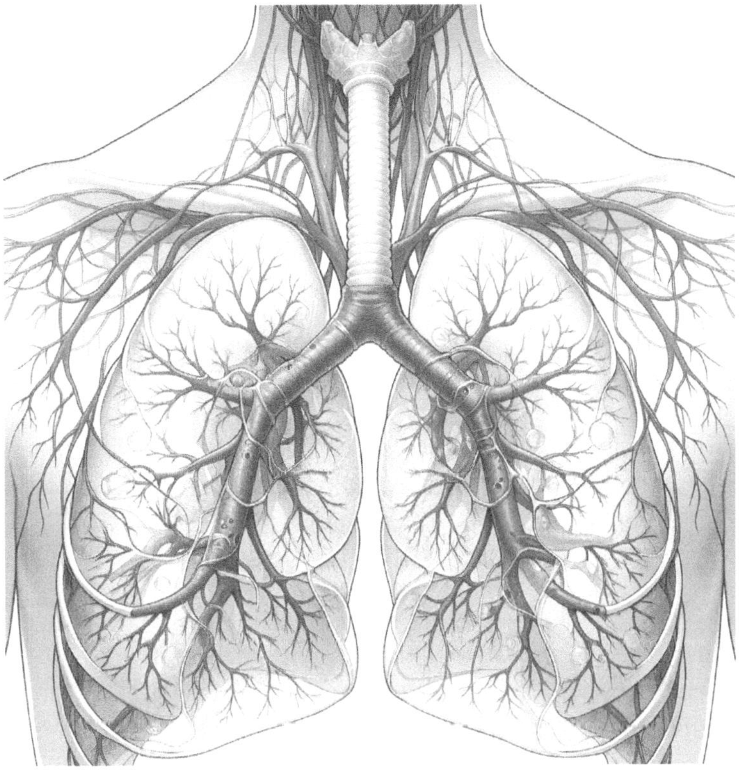

ANATOMY OF THE PULMONARY SYSTEM

The pulmonary system comprises several key structures, each playing a crucial role in the process of respiration.

1. ***Nasal Cavity and Pharynx***

   Breathing begins in the nasal cavity, where air is warmed, moistened, and filtered. The pharynx, a muscular tube, serves as a pathway for both air and food.

2. ***Larynx and Trachea***

   The larynx, or voice box, is located at the top of the trachea and is crucial for speech. The trachea, or windpipe, is a tube that connects the larynx to the bronchi.

3. ***Bronchi and Bronchioles***

   The trachea divides into two main bronchi, each leading to a lung. These bronchi further branch into smaller bronchioles throughout the lungs.

4. ***Lungs and Alveoli***

The lungs are the primary organs of the respiratory system. Within the lungs, bronchioles end in clusters of tiny air sacs called alveoli, where gas exchange occurs.

PHYSIOLOGY OF THE PULMONARY SYSTEM

The physiology of the pulmonary system involves the process of breathing, which can be divided into two phases: inhalation and exhalation.

1. ***Inhalation***

During inhalation, the diaphragm and intercostal muscles contract, expanding the chest cavity and reducing the pressure inside the lungs, drawing in air.

2. ***Gas exchange***

In the alveoli, oxygen from the inhaled air passes through the alveolar walls into the blood in the surrounding capillaries. Simultaneously, carbon dioxide from the blood is expelled into the alveoli.

3. ***Exhalation***

Exhalation is primarily a passive process where the diaphragm and intercostal muscles relax, causing the chest cavity to decrease in size and push air out of the lungs.

THE ROLE OF BLOOD IN THE PULMONARY SYSTEM

The pulmonary system is closely linked with the circulatory system. Oxygenated blood is transported from the lungs to the heart, which then pumps it throughout the body. Deoxygenated blood returns to the lungs for reoxygenation.

DISEASES AND DISORDERS OF THE PULMONARY SYSTEM

Various diseases can affect the pulmonary system, including asthma, chronic obstructive pulmonary disease (COPD), pneumonia, and lung cancer. These conditions can significantly impair respiratory function.

The pulmonary system plays a crucial role in maintaining life by ensuring the continuous exchange of oxygen and carbon dioxide. Understanding its anatomy and physiology is essential for comprehending how our bodies function and for diagnosing and treating respiratory diseases.

TASK 1: FILL IN THE BLANKS

1. Air first enters the respiratory system through the __________ cavity.
2. The __________, also known as the voice box, is crucial for speech.
3. The trachea divides into two main branches called the __________.
4. Small air sacs in the lungs where gas exchange occurs are called __________.

5. The process of breathing can be divided into two phases: __________ and __________.

6. During inhalation, the __________ muscle contracts, expanding the chest cavity.

7. __________ from the air passes through the alveolar walls into the blood in the capillaries.

8. __________ is the primary organ of the respiratory system.

9. Conditions like asthma and COPD affect the __________ system.

TASK 2: LET'S TALK

Nurse 1: Good morning, Mr. Thompson. I'm Nurse Miller, and this is Nurse Johnson. We're here to discuss your asthma management plan.

Patient (Mr. Thompson): Good morning. I've been really worried about my asthma lately.

Nurse 2 (Nurse Johnson): Understandably so, Mr. Thompson. Asthma can be challenging, but with the right management, many people live full, active lives.

Mr. Thompson: That's reassuring to hear. I just don't know much about how to manage it.

Nurse 1: Let's start with the basics. Asthma is a condition where your airways become inflamed and narrow, making breathing difficult. It's part of what we call the pulmonary system, which is vital for gas exchange in your body.

Nurse 2: Exactly. And remember, the lungs are the primary organs in this system. They contain tiny air sacs called alveoli where oxygen enters your blood.

Mr. Thompson: So, how do we treat it?

Nurse 1: Treatment usually involves inhalers. There are two types: a reliever inhaler for immediate relief during an asthma attack, and a preventer inhaler, used daily to keep inflammation down.

Nurse 2: It's like how the nasal cavity filters and warms air. Your inhaler delivers medicine directly to your lungs to reduce inflammation and ease breathing.

Mr. Thompson: I see. How else can I manage my asthma?

Nurse 1: Avoiding triggers is key. Common triggers include pollen, dust, smoke, and even stress.

Nurse 2: Also, regular check-ups are important. Asthma can change over time, so we need to monitor your lung function and adjust treatment as needed.

Mr. Thompson: Can I still exercise?

Nurse 1: Absolutely, exercise is good for lung health. Just be mindful of your limits and have your reliever inhaler on hand.

Nurse 2: And remember, we're here to support you. Managing asthma is a team effort.

Mr. Thompson: Thank you both. I feel much more informed and confident about managing my asthma now.

Nurse 1: You're welcome, Mr. Thompson. If you have any questions or concerns, don't hesitate to reach out to us.

Nurse 2: Yes, we're always here to help. Take care, and remember to stick to your management plan.

TASK 3: DO YOU REMEMBER?

1. **What is another name for the pulmonary system?**

2. **Where does the process of breathing begin in the respiratory system?**

3. **What is the function of the larynx in the respiratory system?**

4. **Into what two main branches does the trachea divide?**

5. **What are the small air sacs in the lungs where gas exchange occurs called?**

6. **Name the two phases of the breathing process.**

7. **Which muscle contracts during inhalation to expand the chest cavity?**

8. **What gas passes from the air into the blood in the capillaries during gas exchange?**

9. **What are the primary organs of the respiratory system?**

10. **Name two conditions, besides asthma, that can affect the pulmonary system.**

11. **What are the two types of inhalers commonly used in asthma treatment?**

12. **What role do the nasal cavity and pharynx play in the respiratory process?**

13. **How can asthma patients avoid triggering their symptoms?**

14. **Why are regular check-ups important for asthma patients?**

15. **Can people with asthma still engage in exercise, and what precaution should they take?**

TASK 4: LATIN AND GREEK TIME

1. **Pulmonary**
   - Derived from the Latin word "pulmonarius," meaning of the lungs.
2. **Respiratory**
   - Comes from the Latin word "respirare," meaning to breathe.
3. **Anatomy**
   - Derived from the Greek word "anatomia" (ἀνατομία), meaning dissection.
4. **Pharynx**
   - Comes from the Greek word "pharynx" (φάρυγξ), meaning throat.
5. **Larynx**

- Derived from the Greek word "laryngos" (λάρυγγος), meaning throat or upper windpipe.

6. **Trachea**
    - Comes from the Greek word "trachys" (τραχύς), meaning rough.
7. **Bronchi**
    - Derived from the Greek word "bronchos" (βρόγχος), meaning windpipe.
8. **Bronchioles**
    - A diminutive form of bronchi, adding "-ole" as a small version of the bronchi.
9. **Alveoli**
    - Comes from the Latin word "alveolus," meaning small cavity or pit.
10. **Physiology**
    - Derived from the Greek words "physis" (φύσις), meaning nature, and "logia" (λογία), meaning study of.
11. **Inhalation**
    - Comes from the Latin word "inhalare," meaning to breathe into.
12. **Exhalation**
    - Derived from the Latin word "exhalare," meaning to breathe out.
13. **Diaphragm**
    - Comes from the Greek word "diaphragma" (διάφραγμα), meaning partition.
14. **Intercostal**
    - *Inter-* comes from the Latin word "inter," meaning between.
    - *Costal* comes from the Latin word "costa," meaning rib.
15. **Circulatory**
    - Derived from the Latin word "circulatus," meaning forming a circle.
16. **Asthma**
    - Comes from the Greek word "asthma" (ἄσθμα), meaning panting or gasping.

17. **Pneumonia**

- Derived from the Greek word "pneumon" (πνεύμων), meaning lung.

18. **Oxygen**

- Comes from the Greek words "oxys" (ὀξύς), meaning sharp, and "genes" (γενής), meaning producer.

19. **Carbon Dioxide**

- *Carbon* comes from the Latin word "carbo," meaning charcoal.
- *Dioxide* combines "di-" (two) from Greek and "oxide," from the French "oxyde," meaning oxygen compound.

TASK 5: MAKE A CHOICE

1. What is the primary function of the pulmonary system?

A) Digestion of food

B) Circulation of blood

C) Exchange of oxygen and carbon dioxide

D) Filtration of waste products

2. Where does the process of breathing begin in the pulmonary system?

A) Larynx B) Trachea C) Nasal cavity D) Bronchi

3. The pharynx serves as a pathway for:

A) Oxygen only B) Carbon dioxide only

C) Both air and food D) Blood flow

4. What is the role of the larynx in the respiratory system?

A) Gas exchange B) Filtering air

C) Speech production D) Blood oxygenation

5. The trachea connects the larynx to the:

A) Heart B) Lungs C) Bronchi D) Alveoli

6. What is the primary function of the bronchi in the pulmonary system?

A) Transporting blood B) Connecting to the lungs

C) Producing mucus D) Absorbing oxygen

7. Alveoli are important for:

A) Warming the air B) Gas exchange

C) Filtering debris D) Producing vocal sounds

8. During inhalation, what happens to the diaphragm?

A) It contracts and expands the chest cavity

B) It relaxes and decreases the chest cavity

C) It stays neutral

D) It filters the air

9. Where does the exchange of oxygen and carbon dioxide occur in the lungs?

A) Bronchi B) Trachea C) Alveoli D) Larynx

10. What is the primary action during exhalation?

A) The diaphragm contracts

B) Air is drawn into the lungs

C) The chest cavity increases in size

D) The diaphragm and intercostal muscles relax

11. How is the pulmonary system linked with the circulatory system?

A) Through nerve connections

B) By transporting oxygenated blood

C) Through digestive processes

D) By filtering waste from blood

12. What is a common disease that affects the pulmonary system?

A) Diabetes B) Asthma C) Arthritis D) Hepatitis

13. What is the primary role of the nasal cavity in respiration?

A) Cooling the air

B) Producing sound

C) Moistening and warming the air

D) Pumping air to the lungs

14. The process of gas exchange in the lungs is essential for:

A) Digesting food B) Muscle contraction

C) Sustaining life D) Blood circulation

15. Chronic obstructive pulmonary disease (COPD) primarily impairs:

A) Kidney function B) Liver function

C) Respiratory function D) Heart function

Chapter 10: The Digestive Process and System: An Essential Guide

The digestive system is a complex and vital part of the human body, playing a crucial role in breaking down food, absorbing nutrients, and eliminating waste. Understanding the digestive process helps in appreciating how our body utilizes food for energy, growth, and cell repair.

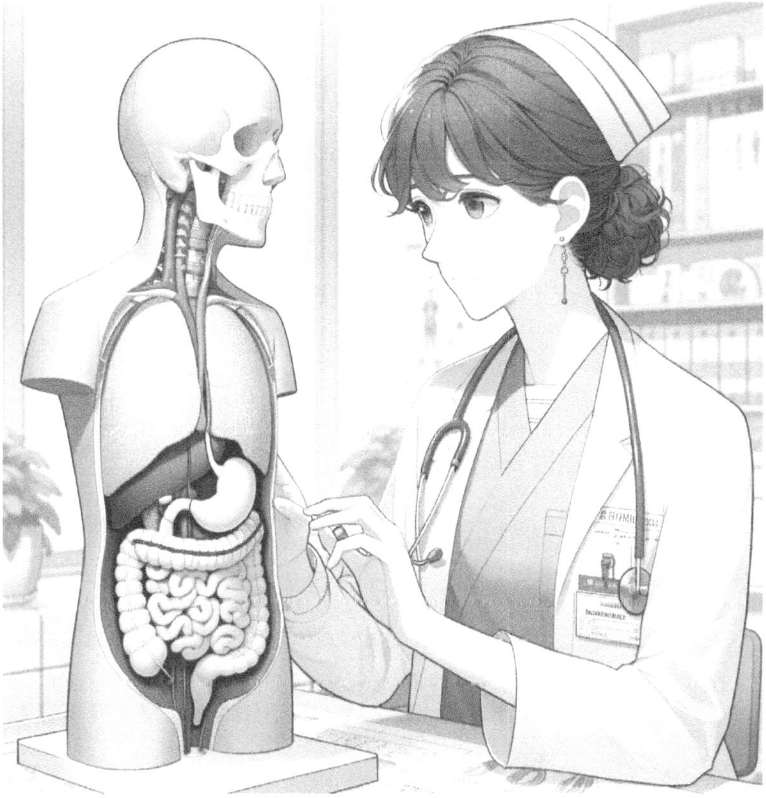

THE JOURNEY OF FOOD: FROM INGESTION TO DIGESTION

MOUTH: THE STARTING POINT

Digestion begins in the mouth. Chewing breaks down food into smaller pieces, while salivary glands secrete saliva containing enzymes like amylase, starting the breakdown of carbohydrates.

ESOPHAGUS: THE FOOD CONDUIT

Swallowed food travels down the oesophagus, a muscular tube connecting the mouth to the stomach. The process of moving food along this tube is called peristalsis.

STOMACH: THE CHEMICAL MIXER

The stomach is a muscular organ that further breaks down food using stomach acid (hydrochloric acid) and enzymes like pepsin, which starts protein digestion. The stomach churns food into a semi-liquid state, called chyme.

SMALL INTESTINE: THE NUTRIENT ABSORBER

Most nutrient absorption occurs in the small intestine. It receives chyme from the stomach, along with bile from the liver and digestive enzymes from the pancreas. These substances work together to break down fats, carbohydrates, and proteins into absorbable units: fatty acids, simple sugars, and amino acids, respectively.

LIVER AND PANCREAS: VITAL ACCESSORY ORGANS

The liver produces bile, crucial for fat digestion and absorption. The pancreas produces enzymes that break down carbohydrates, proteins, and fats. It also secretes bicarbonate to neutralize stomach acid in the small intestine.

LARGE INTESTINE (COLON): WATER ABSORPTION AND WASTE FORMATION

In the large intestine, water and electrolytes are absorbed from the remaining indigestible food matter, forming stool. Beneficial bacteria in the colon aid in this process and contribute to gut health.

RECTUM AND ANUS: THE END LINE

The rectum stores faeces until they are expelled from the body through the anus, completing the digestive process.

THE DIGESTIVE PROCESS: A DETAILED OVERVIEW

1. **Ingestion**: The intake of food.
2. **Mechanical Digestion**: Physical breakdown of food, such as chewing.
3. **Chemical Digestion**: Enzymatic breakdown of food into smaller molecules.
4. **Absorption**: Nutrients from food are absorbed into the bloodstream from the small intestine.
5. **Assimilation**: Absorbed nutrients are transported to different parts of the body for use.
6. **Excretion**: Elimination of indigestible substances as feces.

COMMON DIGESTIVE DISORDERS

The digestive system can be affected by various disorders, such as acid reflux, ulcers, irritable bowel syndrome (IBS), inflammatory bowel disease (IBD), and food intolerances. These conditions can impact the quality of life and require medical attention for management.

The digestive system is a remarkable mechanism, efficiently converting food into essential nutrients. A balanced diet and healthy lifestyle choices contribute significantly to the optimal functioning of this system. Understanding how the digestive system works is not only fascinating but also crucial for recognizing the importance of good nutrition and early detection of digestive disorders.

TASK 1: FILL IN THE BLANKS

1. Digestion begins in the _______, where food is broken down mechanically and mixed with _______.
2. The oesophagus uses _______ to move food from the mouth to the _______.
3. In the stomach, food is mixed with _______ acid and the enzyme _______ to start the digestion of proteins.
4. The majority of nutrient absorption occurs in the _______ intestine.
5. The _______ produces bile, which is essential for fat digestion, while the _______ produces various digestive enzymes.
6. The large intestine, or _______, is primarily involved in the absorption of _______ and the formation of stool.
7. The _______ stores faeces before they are expelled through the _______.
8. The process of ingesting food is known as _______.
9. _______ digestion refers to the enzymatic breakdown of food into smaller molecules.
10. Common digestive disorders include acid _______, ulcers, and irritable bowel _______.

TASK 2: LET'S TALK

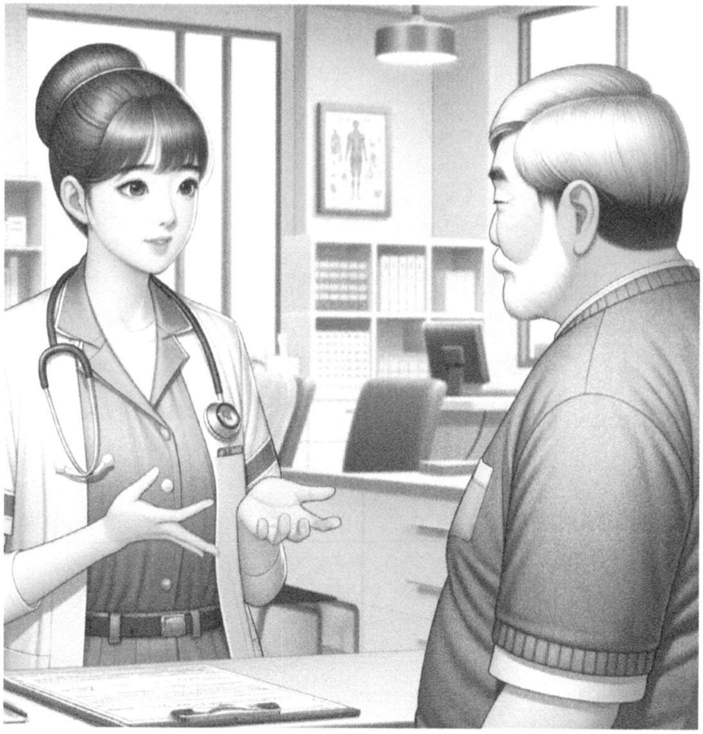

Sarah: Good morning, Tom. How are you feeling today?

Tom: Hi, Sarah. I've been better. My stomach has been bothering me a lot lately.

Sarah: I'm sorry to hear that. Let's talk about your diet and eating habits. How do you typically eat your meals?

Tom: I usually eat pretty quickly, especially when I'm busy. I don't really chew my food much.

Sarah: That might be part of the problem. It's important to chew your food thoroughly. Chewing not only breaks down the food but also mixes it with saliva, which starts the digestion process. Eating too fast can lead to indigestion.

Tom: I didn't realize that. I guess I should slow down and chew more.

Sarah: Exactly. Also, how's your intake of fruits and vegetables?

Tom: To be honest, not great. I don't eat many vegetables.

Sarah: Increasing your intake of vegetables can help with your digestion. They're high in dietary fibre, which is essential for preventing constipation. Fibre helps keep the digestive system moving and can improve overall gut health.

Tom: I've had issues with constipation too, so that makes sense. I'll try to include more vegetables in my diet.

Sarah: That's a good start. It's also helpful to drink plenty of water throughout the day, as hydration plays a key role in digestion and preventing constipation.

Tom: I'll work on that. I usually don't drink much water either.

Sarah: Try carrying a water bottle with you. It can be a good reminder to drink regularly. And when you change your diet to include more fibre, increasing your water intake is even more important.

Tom: Got it. Thanks for the advice, Sarah. I'll start making these changes and see if it helps.

Sarah: You're welcome, Tom. Remember, small changes can make a big difference. If you have any more discomfort or questions, don't hesitate to reach out.

TASK 3: DO YOU UNDERSTAND?

1. **Why does the nurse, Sarah, suggest that Tom should chew his food more thoroughly?**

____

____

____

2. **What is the main reason Tom is experiencing indigestion, according to the nurse?**

____

____

____

3. **How does Sarah link Tom's diet to his constipation issue?**

____

____

____

4. **What dietary change does Sarah recommend to Tom to help with his digestion?**

____

____

____

5. **Why is increasing water intake important when adding more fibre to the diet?**

6. **What practical tip does Sarah give Tom to help him remember to drink more water?**

7. **How does Tom typically eat his meals, and how is this contributing to his digestive issues?**

8. **What does Sarah imply about the role of dietary fibre in gut health?**

9. **What does Tom agree to do to improve his digestion and address his constipation?**

10. **What does Sarah suggest as a general approach to making dietary changes for better digestion?**

TASK 4: LATIN AND GREEK TIME

1. **Digestive**
    - Derived from the Latin word "digestivus," meaning pertaining to digestion.
2. **Nutrients**
    - Comes from the Latin word "nutrire," meaning to nourish.
3. **Mouth**
    - Comes from the Old English word "mūþ," not directly from Latin or Greek.
4. **Salivary**
    - Derived from the Latin word "saliva," meaning saliva.
5. **Amylase**
    - Comes from the Greek word "amylon" (ἄμυλον), meaning starch.
6. **Esophagus**
    - Derived from the Greek word "oisophagos" (οἰσοφάγος), meaning gullet.
7. **Peristalsis**
    - Comes from the Greek words "peri" (περί), meaning around, and "stalsis" (στάλσις), meaning constriction.
8. **Stomach**
    - Comes from the Greek word "stomachos" (στόμαχος), meaning mouth, gullet.
9. **Pepsin**
    - Derived from the Greek word "pepsis" (πέψις), meaning digestion.
10. **Chyme**
    - Comes from the Greek word "chymos" (χυμός), meaning juice.
11. **Intestine**
    - Derived from the Latin word "intestinum," meaning internal.
12. **Bile**
    - Comes from the Latin word "bilis," meaning bile.

13. **Pancreas**

- Derived from the Greek words "pan" (πᾶν), meaning all, and "kreas" (κρέας), meaning flesh.

14. **Bicarbonate**

- *Bi-* comes from the Latin "bis," meaning twice.
- *Carbonate* comes from the Latin "carbonatus," meaning carbonated.

15. **Colon**

- Comes from the Greek word "kolon" (κόλον), meaning large intestine.

16. **Rectum**

- Derived from the Latin word "rectum," meaning straight.

17. **Anus**

- Comes from the Latin word "anus," meaning ring, anus.

18. **Ingestion**

- Derived from the Latin word "ingestio," meaning to throw into.

19. **Assimilation**

- Comes from the Latin word "assimilare," meaning to make similar.

20. **Excretion**

- Derived from the Latin word "excretio," meaning separation.

21. **Ulcers**

- Comes from the Latin word "ulcus," meaning sore, ulcer.

22. **Irritable Bowel Syndrome (IBS)**

- *Irritable* comes from the Latin "irritabilis," meaning easily excited.
- *Bowel* comes from the Old English "būgel," not directly from Latin or Greek.
- *Syndrome* comes from the Greek word "syndromē" (συνδρομή), meaning concurrence.

23. **Inflammatory Bowel Disease (IBD)**

- *Inflammatory* comes from the Latin "inflammare," meaning to set on fire.

- *Bowel* and *Disease* as above.

TASK 5: MAKE A CHOICE

1. What is the primary function of the digestive system?

   A) Circulating blood

   B) Producing hormones

   C) Breaking down food and absorbing nutrients

   D) Filtering waste from the blood

2. Where does the digestion process begin?

   A) Stomach B) Esophagus C) Mouth D) Small intestine

3. What role do salivary glands play in digestion?

   A) Secrete saliva containing enzymes for fat digestion

   B) Produce acids for protein breakdown

   C) Secrete saliva containing enzymes for carbohydrate breakdown

   D) Absorb nutrients

4. The esophagus functions primarily as:

   A) A digestive organ that breaks down food

   B) A conduit for moving food from the mouth to the stomach

   C) The primary site for nutrient absorption

   D) A storage organ for food

5. What is the main function of the stomach in digestion?

A) Absorbing nutrients

B) Producing bile

C) Breaking down food using acid and enzymes

D) Filtering blood

6. Where does most nutrient absorption occur?

A) Large intestine B) Stomach

C) Liver D) Small intestine

7. What is the role of the liver in digestion?

A) Producing digestive enzymes

B) Producing bile for fat digestion

C) Breaking down carbohydrates

D) Absorbing water

8. The large intestine is primarily responsible for:

A) Absorbing water and forming stool

B) Digesting proteins

C) Producing digestive enzymes

D) Secreting bile

9. What is the final stage of the digestive process?

A) Nutrient absorption in the small intestine

B) Excretion of indigestible substances as feces

C) Breakdown of food in the stomach

D) Enzyme secretion by the pancreas

10. Common digestive disorders include:

A) Asthma and bronchitis

B) Ulcers and irritable bowel syndrome

C) Hypertension and diabetes

D) Osteoporosis and arthritis

Chapter 11: The Cardio Vascular System - Part 1

The cardiovascular system, an intricate network comprising the heart, blood vessels, and blood, is indispensable for sustaining life. This system's primary function is to maintain a continuous flow of blood throughout the body, thereby facilitating oxygen and nutrient delivery and waste removal. A deeper understanding of its anatomy and functions reveals the complexity and efficiency of this vital system.

HEART: THE CENTRAL PUMPING ORGAN

The heart, a muscular organ nestled in the thoracic cavity between the lungs, is the powerhouse of the cardiovascular system. It operates as a pump, driving the circulation of blood.

HEART ANATOMY:

- **Chambers**: The heart has four chambers – two atria (upper chambers) and two ventricles (lower chambers). The right atrium and ventricle manage deoxygenated blood, while the left atrium and ventricle handle oxygenated blood.
- **Valves**: The heart comprises four main valves:
    - The tricuspid valve separates the right atrium and ventricle.
    - The pulmonary valve controls blood flow from the right ventricle to the lungs.
    - The mitral valve separates the left atrium and ventricle.
    - The aortic valve opens from the left ventricle to the aorta.

CARDIAC CYCLE:

Each heartbeat involves a sequence of contraction (systole) and relaxation (diastole). During systole, the ventricles contract, pumping blood into the arteries. Diastole sees the heart muscle relax, allowing the chambers to fill with blood.

BLOOD VESSELS: THE EXTENSIVE NETWORK

ARTERIES:

Arteries transport oxygen-rich blood from the heart to the body. They have thick, elastic walls to withstand the high pressure of blood being pumped by the heart. The aorta, the main artery, branches into smaller arteries, delivering blood to various organs.

VEINS:

Veins carry deoxygenated blood back to the heart. They have valves to prevent blood backflow and thinner walls compared to arteries. The superior and inferior vena cava are the largest veins, draining blood into the right atrium of the heart.

CAPILLARIES:

These are the smallest blood vessels where the exchange of oxygen, nutrients, and waste products occurs between blood and tissues. They connect the arterial and venous systems.

BLOOD: THE TRANSPORT MEDIUM

Blood is composed of red blood cells, white blood cells, platelets, and plasma. It carries essential substances like oxygen, nutrients, and hormones, and is pivotal in immune function and homeostasis.

CIRCULATORY PATHWAYS:

SYSTEMIC CIRCULATION:

This pathway carries oxygenated blood from the left side of the heart to the body's tissues and returns deoxygenated blood to the right side of the heart.

PULMONARY CIRCULATION:

It transports deoxygenated blood from the right side of the heart to the lungs for oxygenation and back to the left side of the heart.

CARDIOVASCULAR HEALTH AND DISEASES

Maintaining cardiovascular health is critical. Common diseases affecting this system include:

- **Hypertension**: Elevated blood pressure can lead to heart and blood vessel damage.
- **Atherosclerosis**: Buildup of plaques in the arterial walls, potentially leading to heart attacks and strokes.
- **Coronary Artery Disease**: Narrowing of the coronary arteries, reducing blood flow to the heart muscle.
- **Arrhythmias**: Abnormal heart rhythms that can affect the heart's efficiency.

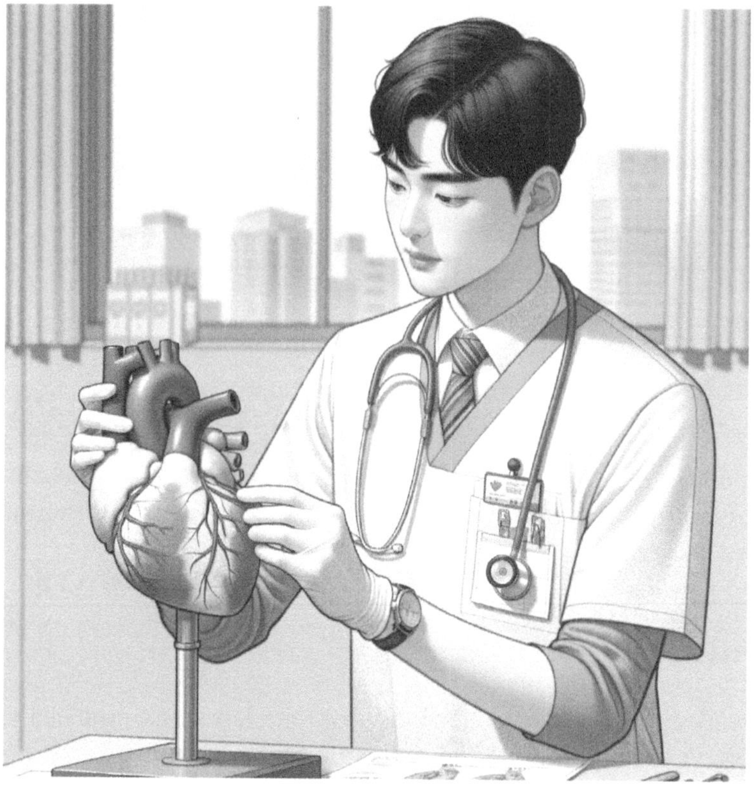

The cardiovascular system's efficient functioning is essential for life. Its complex anatomy and multifaceted roles underscore the importance of heart and blood vessel health. Lifestyle choices, along with regular healthcare, play a pivotal role in maintaining the optimal functioning of this vital system.

TASK 1: FILL IN THE BLANKS

1. The ________ system consists of the heart, ________ vessels, and blood, crucial for circulating blood throughout the body.
2. The heart is located in the ________ cavity and functions as a ________.
3. The heart has four chambers: two ________ and two ________.
4. The four main valves of the heart include the tricuspid, pulmonary, ________, and aortic valves.
5. The ________ cycle consists of two phases: systole (contraction) and diastole (________).
6. ________ transport oxygen-rich blood from the heart to the rest of the body and have thick, ________ walls.
7. ________ return deoxygenated blood back to the heart and are equipped with ________ to prevent backflow.

8. Capillaries are the site of exchange of oxygen, ________, and waste between blood and tissues.

9. Blood is made up of red and white blood cells, ________, and plasma.

10. In systemic circulation, oxygenated blood is carried from the ________ side of the heart to the body's tissues.

11. Pulmonary circulation moves deoxygenated blood from the ________ side of the heart to the lungs for oxygenation.

12. Common cardiovascular diseases include hypertension, atherosclerosis, coronary artery disease, and ________.

TASK 2: LET'S TALK

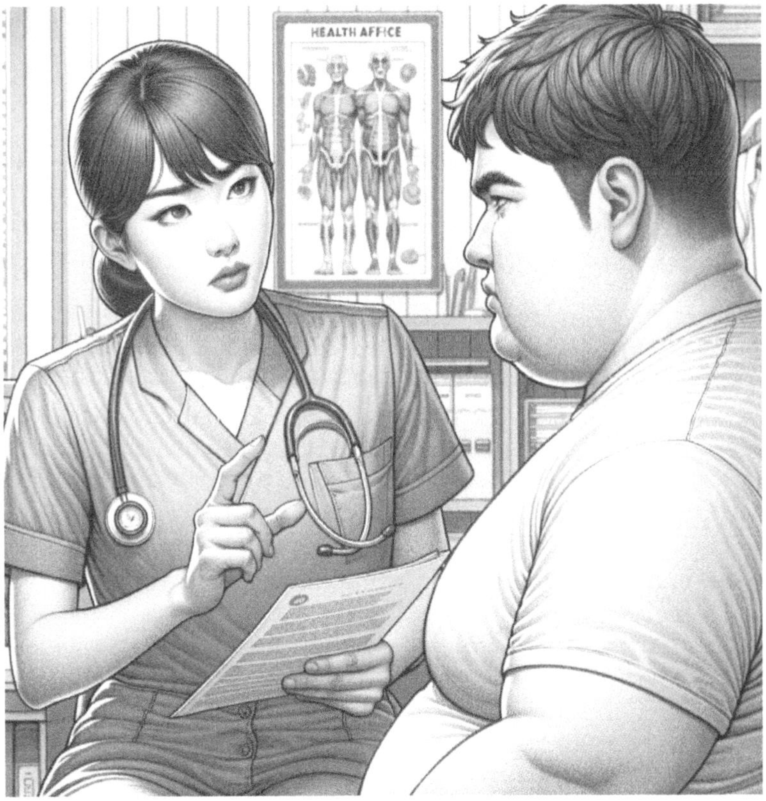

Lisa: Good morning, Mark. I've reviewed your test results and would like to discuss your cardiovascular health.

Mark: Hi, Lisa. I'm a bit anxious. What did the tests show?

Lisa: Your tests indicate that you have hypertension, which is high blood pressure. It's a common issue, but it needs to be managed carefully to avoid further complications.

Mark: Hypertension? I didn't expect that. What does this mean for me?

Lisa: Hypertension means that the force of the blood against your artery walls is consistently too high. It can lead to more serious conditions, like heart disease or stroke, if not managed properly.

Mark: So, what should I do?

Lisa: Firstly, it's important to make some lifestyle changes. Regular physical activity can significantly help in lowering blood pressure. Also, adopting a heart-healthy diet that's low in salt, saturated fats, and cholesterol is crucial.

Mark: I see. I guess I need to be more careful about what I eat and start exercising.

Lisa: Exactly. It's also important to monitor your blood pressure regularly. We can help you learn how to do this at home.

Mark: Will I need medication?

Lisa: That depends on various factors, including the severity of your hypertension. Medications can be very effective in managing high blood pressure, especially when combined with lifestyle changes.

Mark: I understand. Is there anything else I should know?

Lisa: Yes, it's vital to manage stress, as it can also impact your blood pressure. Techniques like deep breathing can be beneficial.

Mark: Okay, I will definitely give those a try. Thank you, Lisa, for explaining everything.

Lisa: You're welcome, Mark. Remember, managing hypertension is a team effort. We'll schedule regular check-ups to monitor your progress and adjust the treatment plan as needed.

TASK 3: DO YOU REMEMBER?

1. **What are the main components of the cardiovascular system?**

____

____

____

2. **Where is the heart located in the human body?**

____

____

____

3. **How many chambers does the heart have, and what are they called?**

4. **Name the four main valves of the heart.**

5. **What are the two phases of the cardiac cycle?**

6. **What type of blood do arteries carry, and what is unique about their walls?**

7. **What is the function of veins, and what feature do they have to aid this function?**

8. **What occurs in the capillaries?**

9. **What four main components make up blood?**

10. **What is the difference between systemic circulation and pulmonary circulation?**

11. **What cardiovascular condition was Mark diagnosed with?**

12. **List some lifestyle changes recommended for managing hypertension.**

13. **Why is regular physical activity important for cardiovascular health?**

14. **How can stress impact blood pressure?**

15. **What should Mark do to regularly monitor his condition at home?**

TASK 4: LATIN AND GREEK TIME

1. **Cardiovascular**
   - *Cardio-*: From the Greek word "kardia" (καρδιά), meaning heart.
   - *Vascular*: From the Latin word "vasculum," meaning small vessel.
2. **Thoracic**
   - From the Greek word "thorax" (θώραξ), meaning chest, breastplate.
3. **Atria**
   - From the Latin word "atrium," meaning an entrance hall.
4. **Ventricles**
   - From the Latin word "ventriculus," meaning a small belly or cavity.
5. **Tricuspid Valve**
   - *Tri-*: From the Latin word "tres," meaning three.
   - *Cuspid*: From the Latin word "cuspis," meaning point.
6. **Pulmonary**
   - From the Latin word "pulmonarius," meaning of the lungs.
7. **Mitral Valve**
   - From the Latin word "mitra," meaning a turban or headdress, referring to the valve's shape.
8. **Aortic**
   - From the Greek word "aortē" (ἀορτή), meaning great artery.
9. **Systole**
   - From the Greek word "systolē" (συστολή), meaning contraction.
10. **Diastole**

- From the Greek word "diastolē" (διαστολή), meaning dilation.

11. **Arteries**

- From the Greek word "arteria" (ἀρτηρία), meaning windpipe, artery.

12. **Veins**

- From the Latin word "vena," meaning vein.

13. **Capillaries**

- From the Latin word "capillaris," meaning hair-like.

14. **Systemic**

- From the Greek word "systema" (σύστημα), meaning whole compounded of several parts.

15. **Pulmonary Circulation**

- *Pulmonary*: As above.
- *Circulation*: From the Latin word "circulatio," meaning going around.

16. **Hypertension**

- *Hyper-*: From the Greek word "hyper" (ὑπέρ), meaning over, above.

17. **Atherosclerosis**

- *Athero-*: From the Greek word "athēra" (ἀθήρα), meaning porridge (referring to the plaque's consistency).
- *Sclerosis*: From the Greek word "sklerosis" (σκλήρωσις), meaning hardening.

18. **Coronary**

- From the Latin word "coronarius," meaning of a crown (referring to the way these arteries encircle the heart).

19. **Arrhythmias**

- From the Greek words "a-" (ἀ-), meaning not, without, and "rhythmos" (ῥυθμός), meaning rhythm.

TASK 5: MAKE A CHOICE

1. What is the primary function of the cardiovascular system?

A) Digestion of food

B) Regulation of body temperature

C) Continuous flow of blood throughout the body

D) Oxygenation of muscles

2. Where is the heart located?

A) In the abdominal cavity

B) Between the lungs in the thoracic cavity

C) In the lower spine

D) Under the left rib cage

3. How many chambers does the heart have?

A) Two B) Four C) Six D) Eight

4. Which valve separates the right atrium and ventricle?

A) Mitral valve B) Pulmonary valve

C) Aortic valve D) Tricuspid valve

5. What is systole?

A) Relaxation of the heart

B) Contraction of the heart

C) Slowing of the heartbeat

D) Acceleration of the heartbeat

6. What type of blood vessels carry oxygen-rich blood from the heart to the body?

A) Veins B) Arteries C) Capillaries D) Venules

7. What is the main function of veins?

A) To carry deoxygenated blood back to the heart

B) To supply oxygen to the muscles

C) To exchange gases in tissues

D) To regulate blood pressure

8. Capillaries are:

A) The largest blood vessels

B) Involved in the exchange of oxygen and nutrients

C) Only found in the heart

D) Thick-walled vessels

9. Which system does the cardiovascular system work closely with to sustain life?

A) Digestive system B) Respiratory system

C) Nervous system D) Muscular system

10. What is the largest artery in the body?

A) Pulmonary artery B) Aorta

C) Carotid artery D) Femoral artery

11. What is hypertension?

A) Low blood pressure B) High blood pressure

C) Normal blood pressure D) Irregular heart rhythm

12. Atherosclerosis involves the buildup of plaques in which type of blood vessel?

A) Arteries B) Veins C) Capillaries D) Venules

13. What does coronary artery disease affect?

A) The lungs B) The heart muscle

C) The brain D) The liver

14. What is an arrhythmia?

A) A normal heart rhythm B) A blood clot in the heart

C) An abnormal heart rhythm D) A blocked artery

Chapter 12: The Cardio Vascular System- Part 2

The circulatory system, a vital network in the human body, comprises the heart, blood vessels, and blood. It is responsible for transporting nutrients, oxygen, hormones, and waste products throughout the body. This system not only nourishes cells and tissues but also plays a critical role in maintaining homeostasis. However, like any complex system, it is susceptible to various disorders and diseases.

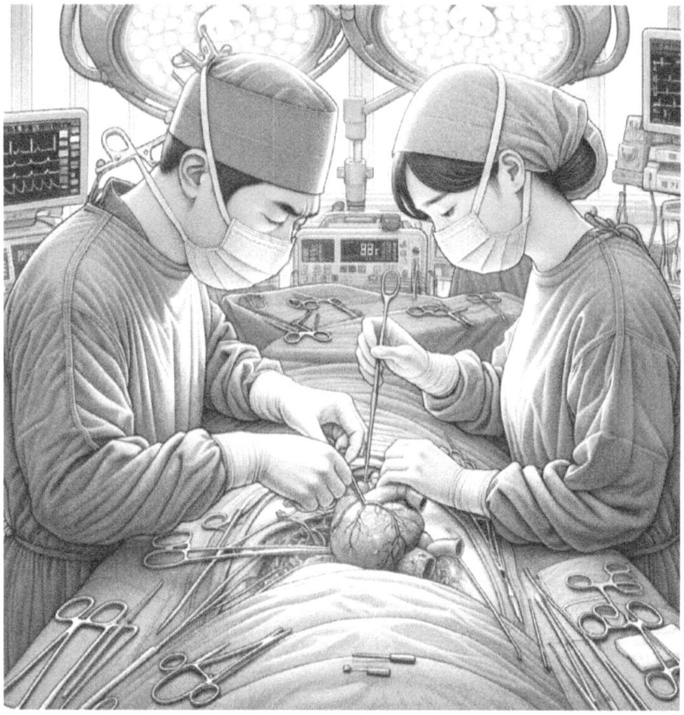

ANATOMY OF THE CIRCULATORY SYSTEM

HEART

The heart, a powerful muscular organ, pumps blood throughout the body. It has four chambers: two atria and two ventricles. The heart's rhythmic contractions maintain blood flow in two distinct circuits: the pulmonary circuit (lungs) and the systemic circuit (rest of the body).

BLOOD VESSELS

The blood vessels include arteries, veins, and capillaries. Arteries carry oxygen-rich blood away from the heart, veins return oxygen-depleted blood back to the heart, and capillaries facilitate the exchange of gases, nutrients, and waste between blood and tissues.

BLOOD

Blood is composed of red blood cells, white blood cells, platelets, and plasma. It plays a vital role in transporting various substances, including oxygen and nutrients, to the cells and removing waste products.

COMMON DISEASES OF THE CIRCULATORY SYSTEM

HYPERTENSION (HIGH BLOOD PRESSURE)

Hypertension is a condition where the blood pressure in the arteries is persistently elevated. Long-term high blood pressure can lead to various health issues, including heart disease, stroke, and kidney failure.

CORONARY ARTERY DISEASE (CAD)

CAD occurs when the coronary arteries, which supply blood to the heart muscle, become hardened and narrowed due to plaque build-up. This can lead to chest pain (angina) and heart attacks.

HEART FAILURE

Heart failure is a condition where the heart cannot pump enough blood to meet the body's needs. It can result from various underlying issues, including coronary artery disease and hypertension.

ARRHYTHMIAS

Arrhythmias are irregular heartbeats. They can manifest as tachycardia (too fast), bradycardia (too slow), or fibrillation (irregular), affecting the heart's efficiency and overall function.

STROKE

A stroke occurs when the blood supply to part of the brain is interrupted or reduced, preventing brain tissue from getting oxygen and nutrients. Strokes can be caused by blocked arteries (ischemic stroke) or leaking or burst blood vessels (hemorrhagic stroke).

PERIPHERAL ARTERY DISEASE (PAD)

PAD is the narrowing of peripheral arteries, typically in the legs, due to atherosclerosis. This can cause leg pain, especially during walking, and can lead to more severe complications.

DEEP VEIN THROMBOSIS (DVT) AND PULMONARY EMBOLISM (PE)

DVT is the formation of a blood clot in a deep vein, usually in the legs. A clot can dislodge and travel to the lungs, causing a pulmonary embolism, a potentially life-threatening condition.

The circulatory system is integral to the functioning of the human body, and its health is essential for overall well-being. Understanding the common diseases associated with the circulatory system can aid in early detection, prevention, and effective management. Regular exercise, a balanced diet, maintaining a healthy weight, and not smoking are critical steps in promoting circulatory system health. Regular medical check-ups and monitoring of blood pressure and cholesterol levels are also key in preventing and managing these common circulatory diseases.

TASK 1: FILL IN THE BLANKS

1. The __________ system consists of the heart, _______ vessels, and blood.

2. The heart is divided into four chambers: two _______ and two ________.

3. Arteries carry _______-rich blood away from the heart, while veins carry _______-depleted blood back.

4. Capillaries are small vessels where the exchange of _______, nutrients, and waste occurs.

5. _________ is a condition of persistently elevated blood pressure in the arteries.

6. _________ Artery Disease is characterized by the hardening and narrowing of coronary arteries.

7. Heart _______ is a condition where the heart can't pump enough blood to meet the body's needs.

8. _________ are types of irregular heartbeats, which can be too fast, too slow, or irregular.

9. A _______ is caused by an interrupted or reduced blood supply to part of the brain.

10. _________ Artery Disease involves the narrowing of peripheral arteries due to atherosclerosis.

11. _______ Vein Thrombosis is the formation of a blood clot in a deep vein, usually in the _______.

12. A clot from DVT can travel to the lungs, causing a _________ Embolism.

TASK 2: LET'S TALK

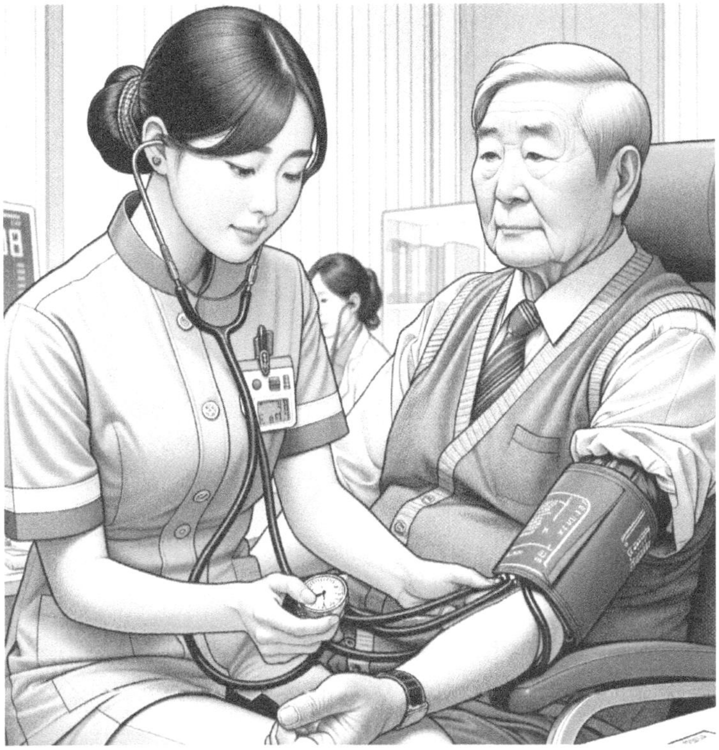

Dr. Jeong: Good morning, Nurse Lee. I've just reviewed Mr. Kim's chart. His symptoms suggest a cardiovascular issue.

Nurse Lee: Good morning, Dr. Jeong. Yes, I was concerned about his elevated blood pressure and shortness of breath. Could it be hypertension?

Dr. Jeong: That's a possibility. Hypertension is often a silent contributor to more serious conditions like coronary artery disease or even heart failure.

Nurse Lee: I see. Mr. Kim mentioned occasional chest pains, especially during physical activity.

Dr. Jeong: That could indicate Coronary Artery Disease. The stress on the heart during physical activity can exacerbate symptoms if the coronary arteries are narrowed.

Nurse Lee: Should we be concerned about the risk of a heart attack?

Dr. Jeong: Definitely. We need to conduct further tests to assess the condition of his heart and arteries. Given his symptoms, an arrhythmia could also be a possibility.

Nurse Lee: Yes, his heart rate did seem irregular during the initial examination. Do you think a stroke could also be a risk factor here?

Dr. Jeong: It's important to consider all possibilities, including a stroke, especially with his history of hypertension. We should monitor his neurological signs closely.

Nurse Lee: What about peripheral artery disease? He mentioned leg pain when walking.

Dr. Jeong: That's a good point, Nurse Lee. We should assess blood flow in his legs. Sometimes, peripheral artery disease can coexist with coronary artery disease.

Nurse Lee: Regarding his treatment plan, should we start with lifestyle modifications?

Dr. Jeong: Absolutely. Lifestyle changes are crucial. We'll need to address his diet, physical activity, and stress management. Medication might also be necessary depending on our findings.

Nurse Lee: I'll prepare the patient for the tests and ensure he understands the importance of these lifestyle changes.

Dr. Jeong: Thank you, Nurse Lee. Let's prioritize a comprehensive cardiovascular assessment for Mr. Kim and go from there.

TASK 3: DO YOU REMEMBER?

1. **What are the primary components of the circulatory system?**

____
____
____

2. **How many chambers does the heart have?**

____
____
____

3. **What is the function of arteries in the circulatory system?**

____
____
____

4. **What role do capillaries play in the circulatory system?**

____
____
____

5. **What condition is indicated by persistently high blood pressure?**

6. **What is Coronary Artery Disease and what does it affect?**

7. **What are potential symptoms of Coronary Artery Disease?**

8. **How can hypertension contribute to the risk of a heart attack?**

9. **What are arrhythmias and why are they a concern in cardiovascular health?**

10. **Why might a stroke be a concern for someone with cardiovascular issues?**

11. **What is Peripheral Artery Disease and what are its symptoms?**

____

____

____

12. **What lifestyle changes are often recommended for managing cardiovascular diseases?**

____

____

____

13. **What type of tests might Dr. Jeong consider for assessing Mr. Kim's heart condition?**

____

____

____

14. **Why is it important to monitor neurological signs in patients with hypertension?**

____

____

____

15. **What did Nurse Lee suggest she would do to help the patient understand the treatment plan?**

____

____

____

TASK 4: LATIN AND GREEK TIME

1. **Cardiovascular**
   - *Cardio-* comes from the Greek word "kardia" (καρδιά), meaning heart.
   - *Vascular* comes from the Latin word "vasculum," meaning small vessel.
2. **Anatomy**

- Derived from the Greek word "anatomia" (ἀνατομία), meaning dissection.

3. **Thoracic**

- Comes from the Greek word "thorax" (θώραξ), meaning breastplate, chest.

4. **Atria**

- Derived from the Latin word "atrium," meaning an entrance hall.

5. **Ventricles**

- Comes from the Latin word "ventriculus," meaning small belly or cavity.

6. **Tricuspid**

- *Tri-* comes from the Latin word "tres," meaning three.
- *Cuspid* comes from the Latin word "cuspis," meaning point.

7. **Pulmonary**

- Derived from the Latin word "pulmonarius," meaning of the lungs.

8. **Mitral**

- Comes from the Latin word "mitra," meaning a turban or headdress, due to its shape.

9. **Aorta**

- Derived from the Greek word "aorte" (ἀορτή), meaning suspension, the great artery.

10. **Arteries**

- Comes from the Greek word "arteria" (ἀρτηρία), meaning windpipe, artery.

11. **Veins**

- Derived from the Latin word "vena," meaning vein.

12. **Capillaries**

- Comes from the Latin word "capillaris," meaning hair-like.

13. **Systole**

- Derived from the Greek word "systolē" (συστολή), meaning contraction.

14. **Diastole**

- Comes from the Greek word "diastolē" (διαστολή), meaning dilation.

15. **Hypertension**

- *Hyper-* comes from the Greek word "hyper" (ὑπέρ), meaning over.
- *Tension* comes from the Latin word "tensio," meaning stretching.

16. **Atherosclerosis**

- *Athero-* comes from the Greek word "athera" (ἀθήρα), meaning porridge (referring to the fatty deposits).
- *Sclerosis* comes from the Greek word "sklerosis" (σκλήρωσις), meaning hardening.

17. **Coronary**

- Derived from the Latin word "coronarius," meaning crown-like.

18. **Arrhythmias**

- *A-* is a prefix meaning not or without.
- *Rhythmias* comes from the Greek word "rhythmos" (ῥυθμός), meaning rhythm.

TASK 5: MAKE A CHOICE

1. What is the primary function of the cardiovascular system?

A) Digestion of food

B) Regulation of body temperature

C) Maintenance of blood flow throughout the body

D) Filtering of waste products

2. Where is the heart located in the human body?

A) Abdominal cavity B) Pelvic cavity

C) Thoracic cavity D) Cranial cavity

3. How many chambers does the heart have?

A) Two B) Three C) Four D) Five

4. The right atrium and ventricle manage:

A) Oxygenated blood B) Deoxygenated blood

C) Nutrients D) Waste products

5. The tricuspid valve separates:

A) The left atrium and ventricle

B) The right atrium and ventricle

C) The two atria

D) The two ventricles

6. What does the pulmonary valve control?

A) Blood flow from the right ventricle to the lungs

B) Blood flow from the left ventricle to the lungs

C) Blood flow from the lungs to the heart

D) Blood flow from the heart to the rest of the body

7. What is the main function of arteries?

A) Transport oxygen-rich blood from the heart to the body

B) Carry deoxygenated blood back to the heart

C) Connect the arterial and venous systems

D) Filter blood

8. What is the primary role of veins in the cardiovascular system?

A) Supply oxygen to the heart

B) Carry oxygen-rich blood to the body

C) Transport deoxygenated blood back to the heart

D) Produce blood cells

9. Capillaries are responsible for:

A) Pumping blood

B) The exchange of oxygen, nutrients, and waste products

C) Carrying blood to the lungs

D) Generating heartbeats

10. Blood is composed of:

A) Only red and white blood cells

B) Only plasma

C) Red blood cells, white blood cells, platelets, and plasma

D) Only platelets and plasma

11. Systemic circulation involves:

A) Carrying oxygenated blood from the right side of the heart to the body

B) Carrying deoxygenated blood from the left side of the heart to the body

C) Carrying oxygenated blood from the left side of the heart to the body

D) Carrying deoxygenated blood from the right side of the heart to the lungs

12. Pulmonary circulation transports blood:

A) From the heart to the rest of the body

B) From the lungs to the rest of the body

C) From the right side of the heart to the lungs

D) From the left side of the heart to the lungs

13. What is hypertension?

A) Low blood pressure

B) Elevated blood pressure

C) Normal blood pressure

D) The absence of blood pressure

14. Atherosclerosis is characterized by:

A) Buildup of plaques in the arterial walls

B) Low levels of oxygen in the blood

C) Increased blood cell production

D) Expansion of the veins

15. What does coronary artery disease result in?

A) Increased blood flow to the brain

B) Narrowing of the coronary arteries

C) Strengthening of the heart muscle

D) Reduction in blood vessel elasticity

Chapter 13: The Lymphatic System

The lymphatic system, an essential part of the immune system, plays a vital role in maintaining bodily fluid levels, absorbing digestive tract fats, and protecting against infections. Comprising a network of lymphatic vessels, lymph nodes, and organs like the spleen and thymus, it works in concert with the circulatory system to keep body fluids in balance and defend against diseases.

ANATOMY OF THE LYMPHATIC SYSTEM

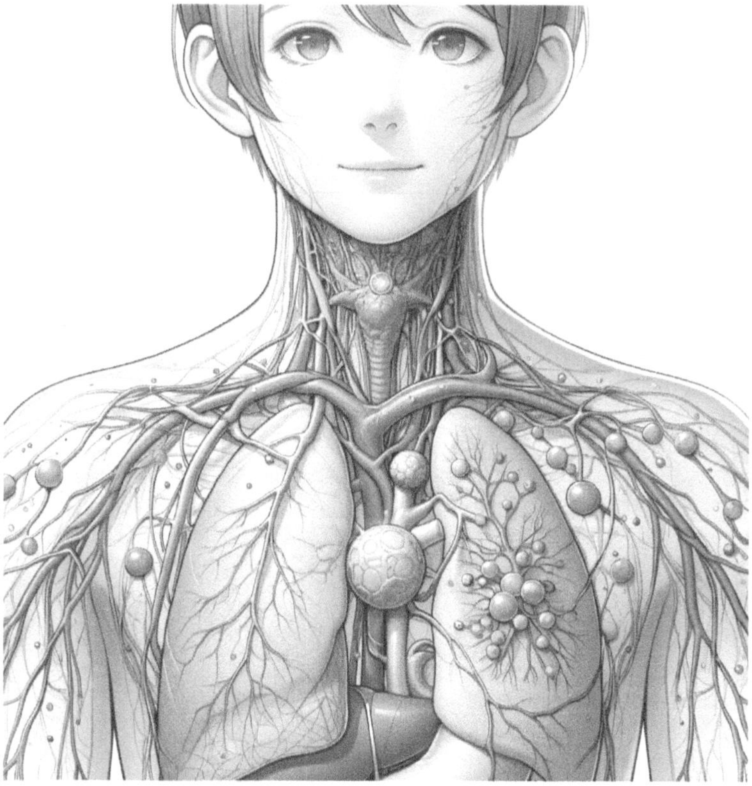

LYMPHATIC VESSELS

These vessels transport lymph, a clear fluid containing white blood cells, especially lymphocytes. Lymphatic vessels begin as small capillaries and merge into larger tubes, transporting lymph back into the bloodstream.

LYMPH NODES

Scattered throughout the body, lymph nodes filter lymph to remove foreign particles. Common areas with concentrated lymph nodes include the neck, armpits, and groin.

SPLEEN

The spleen filters and purifies blood and lymph fluid, removing old or damaged red blood cells. It also helps fight certain kinds of bacteria.

THYMUS

Located in the upper chest, the thymus is the maturation site for T lymphocytes (T cells), a type of white blood cell crucial for adaptive immunity.

TONSILS AND ADENOIDS

These lymphoid tissues in the throat area help protect against pathogens entering the body through the mouth or nose.

FUNCTIONS OF THE LYMPHATIC SYSTEM

1. **Fluid Balance**: The lymphatic system returns excess interstitial fluid to the bloodstream, maintaining fluid balance in the body.
2. **Absorption of Fatty Acids**: It absorbs fatty acids and fats from the digestive system and transports them to the circulatory system.
3. **Immune Responses**: The system is essential for immune surveillance and response. Lymph nodes produce and store cells that help fight infection, including lymphocytes, macrophages, and dendritic cells.

COMMON AILMENTS OF THE LYMPHATIC SYSTEM

LYMPHEDEMA

This occurs when lymph accumulates in tissues, causing swelling, most commonly in the arms and legs. It can result from the removal of or damage to lymph nodes.

LYMPHADENOPATHY

Enlarged lymph nodes, often due to infection, inflammation, or malignancy. This condition can be a sign of various diseases, including infections, autoimmune disorders, or cancers like lymphoma.

LYMPHANGITIS

Inflammation of the lymphatic vessels, typically caused by a bacterial infection. It presents as red streaks on the skin, extending from the infected area.

LYMPHOMA

A type of cancer affecting the lymphatic system, lymphoma involves the uncontrolled growth of lymphocytes. Hodgkin's lymphoma and non-Hodgkin's lymphoma are the two main types.

TONSILLITIS AND ADENOIDITIS

Inflammation of the tonsils and adenoids, usually due to infection. It can cause sore throat, difficulty swallowing, and swollen lymph nodes around the neck.

TASK 1: FILL IN THE BLANKS

1. The ________ system is an essential part of the immune system and maintains ________ balance in the body.
2. Lymphatic vessels transport ________, a clear fluid containing white blood cells.
3. ________ nodes are small structures that filter lymph to remove foreign particles.
4. The ________ filters blood and lymph fluid, removing old red blood cells and helping fight certain bacteria.
5. The ________ is where T lymphocytes mature and is crucial for adaptive immunity.
6. The lymphatic system plays a key role in the absorption of fatty acids from the ________ system.
7. ________ is the condition where lymph accumulates in tissues, causing swelling.
8. Enlarged lymph nodes, a condition known as ________, can indicate infections, autoimmune disorders, or cancers.
9. ________ is the inflammation of the lymphatic vessels, often caused by bacterial infection.
10. ________ is a type of cancer that affects the lymphatic system, with two main types being Hodgkin's and non-Hodgkin's.
11. Inflammation of the tonsils and adenoids is referred to as ________ and ________, respectively.
12. Regular ________ activity, a balanced diet, and good hygiene are essential for maintaining a healthy lymphatic system.

TASK 2: LET'S TALK

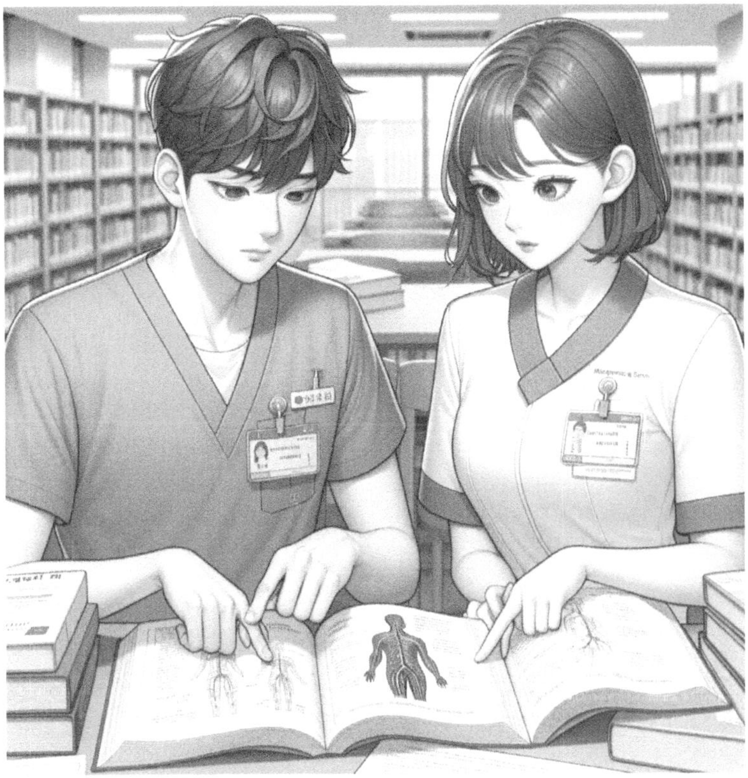

Alex: Hey Mia, are you ready for the lymphatic system exam?

Mia: I think so, Alex. I've been reviewing the notes. The lymphatic system is quite fascinating, isn't it?

Alex: Absolutely. It's amazing how it maintains fluid balance in the body and is part of the immune system. But there's a lot to remember.

Mia: Definitely. Like how the lymphatic vessels carry lymph, which is this fluid containing white blood cells.

Alex: Right, and the lymph nodes are crucial since they filter the lymph. I remember they're located in areas like the neck, armpits, and groin.

Mia: Exactly. And don't forget the spleen and thymus. The spleen filters blood, while the thymus is where T cells mature.

Alex: Oh, yes, the thymus. That's important for adaptive immunity. What about the ailments we need to know?

Mia: Well, there's lymphedema, where lymph accumulates and causes swelling. It's often due to damaged lymph nodes.

Alex: And lymphadenopathy, the enlargement of lymph nodes, which can signal infections or even cancers like lymphoma.

Mia: Lymphoma was a big topic. Remember, there are two types: Hodgkin's and non-Hodgkin's.

Alex: I'm also reviewing lymphangitis, the inflammation of lymphatic vessels. It's typically caused by a bacterial infection.

Mia: That's important. And don't forget tonsillitis and adenoiditis, inflammations due to infections, affecting the throat.

Alex: Right. We also need to know how to keep the lymphatic system healthy – like through regular exercise and good hygiene.

Mia: Definitely. It's all about early detection and management of lymphatic disorders.

Alex: Thanks, Mia. This review session was really helpful. I feel more prepared for the exam now.

Mia: Same here, Alex. Let's ace this test!

TASK 3: DO YOU REMEMBER?

1. **What is the primary function of the lymphatic system?**

____

____

____

2. **What type of fluid do lymphatic vessels transport?**

____

____

____

3. **Where are lymph nodes predominantly located in the body?**

____

____

____

4. **What is the role of the spleen in the lymphatic system?**

5. **Where do T lymphocytes mature in the lymphatic system?**

6. **What is lymphedema and what causes it?**

7. **What does lymphadenopathy indicate about a person's health?**

8. **Name the two main types of lymphoma.**

9. **What is lymphangitis and what typically causes it?**

10. **What are tonsillitis and adenoiditis, and what causes these conditions?**

11. **How can one maintain a healthy lymphatic system?**

12. **What role does the thymus play in immunity?**

13. **Why is the lymphatic system important for fluid balance in the body?**

14. **What type of cells does lymph contain?**

15. **What is the importance of early detection and management of lymphatic disorders?**

TASK 4: LATIN AND GREEK TIME

1. **Lymphatic**

- Derived from the Latin word "lympha," meaning water or clear fluid.

2. **Immune**

- Comes from the Latin word "immunis," meaning exempt or protected.

3. **Vessels**

- Derived from the Latin word "vasculum," meaning small vessel.

4. **Lymph**

- As in lymphatic, from the Latin word "lympha".

5. **Nodes**

- Comes from the Latin word "nodus," meaning knot.

6. **Spleen**

- Derived from the Greek word "splen" (σπλήν), meaning spleen.

7. **Thymus**

- Comes from the Greek word "thymos" (θύμος), meaning thyme (due to its similarity in shape).

8. **Tonsils**

- Derived from the Latin word "tonsilla," meaning almond or tonsil.

9. **Adenoids**

- Comes from the Greek word "aden" (ἀδήν), meaning gland, and "-oid," meaning like or resembling.

10. **Interstitial**

- Derived from the Latin word "interstitium," meaning space or interval.

11. **Macrophages**

- *Macro-* comes from the Greek word "makros" (μακρός), meaning large.
- *-phages* comes from the Greek word "phagein" (φαγεῖν), meaning to eat.

12. **Dendritic**

- Derived from the Greek word "dendron" (δένδρον), meaning tree.

13. **Lymphedema**

- *Lymph-* as in lymphatic.
- *-edema* comes from the Greek word "oidēma" (οἴδημα), meaning swelling.

14. **Lymphadenopathy**

- *Lymphaden-* combines "lympha" from Latin and "aden" (ἀδήν) from Greek, meaning gland.
- *-pathy* comes from the Greek word "pathos" (πάθος), meaning suffering or disease.

15. **Lymphangitis**

- *Lymph-* as in lymphatic.
- *-angitis* comes from the Greek word "angeion" (ἀγγεῖον), meaning vessel, and "-itis," meaning inflammation.

16. **Lymphoma**

- *Lymph-* as in lymphatic.
- *-oma* comes from the Greek word "oma" (ώμα), meaning tumor.

17. **Tonsillitis**

- *Tonsil-* as in tonsils.
- *-itis* indicating inflammation.

18. **Adenoiditis**

- *Adenoid-* as in adenoids.
- *-itis* indicating inflammation.

TASK 5: MAKE A CHOICE

1. What is the primary role of the lymphatic system?

A) Regulating body temperature

B) Maintaining bodily fluid levels

C) Producing red blood cells

D) Breaking down nutrients

2. Lymphatic vessels primarily transport:

A) Red blood cells

B) Platelets

C) Lymph, a clear fluid containing white blood cells

D) Oxygen

3. Lymph nodes function to:

A) Produce lymph

B) Filter lymph and remove foreign particles

C) Transport oxygen

D) Absorb nutrients

4. The spleen plays a crucial role in:

A) Filtering and purifying blood and lymph fluid

B) Producing digestive enzymes

C) Regulating body temperature

D) Absorbing fats

5. The thymus is important for:

A) The maturation of T lymphocytes

B) Filtering lymph

C) Breaking down carbohydrates

D) Producing hormones

6. Tonsils and adenoids help protect against:

A) Pathogens entering through the mouth or nose

B) Blood clots

C) Nutrient deficiencies

D) Temperature fluctuations

7. What is lymphedema characterized by?

A) High lymph production

B) Swelling due to lymph accumulation in tissues

C) Decreased white blood cell count

D) Excessive sweating

8. Lymphadenopathy refers to:

A) Enlarged lymph nodes

B) Inflammation of the lymphatic vessels

C) A type of lymphatic cancer

D) A deficiency in lymph production

9. Lymphangitis is:

A) Inflammation of the lymph nodes

B) A decrease in lymph flow

C) Inflammation of the lymphatic vessels

D) An increase in lymph production

10. Lymphoma is:

A) A benign growth in the lymphatic system

B) Inflammation of lymphatic vessels

C) A type of cancer affecting the lymphatic system

D) Swelling of the lymph nodes

11. Tonsillitis and adenoiditis are:

A) Types of blood disorders

B) Inflammatory conditions of the lymphoid tissues in the throat

C) Cancers of the lymphatic system

D) Disorders related to lymph production

12. What is the function of the fluid balance in the lymphatic system?

A) To regulate body temperature

B) To return excess interstitial fluid to the bloodstream

C) To transport nutrients to cells

D) To produce hormones

13. How do lymphatic vessels begin in the body?

A) As large tubes B) As small capillaries

C) As muscular valves D) As bony structures

14. What is a key function of the immune responses of the lymphatic system?

A) Producing digestive enzymes

B) Regulating blood pressure

C) Fighting infection

D) Absorbing carbohydrates

15. Absorption of fatty acids in the lymphatic system occurs primarily in the:

A) Lungs B) Liver C) Digestive system D) Kidneys

Chapter 14 : Quarantine Matters!

The concept of quarantine, a critical public health measure, has evolved significantly over centuries, adapting to the challenges posed by various infectious diseases. This article explores the historical development of quarantine practices, the implication of biosafety levels, and the establishment of high-level bio-safety laboratories, particularly in East Asia.

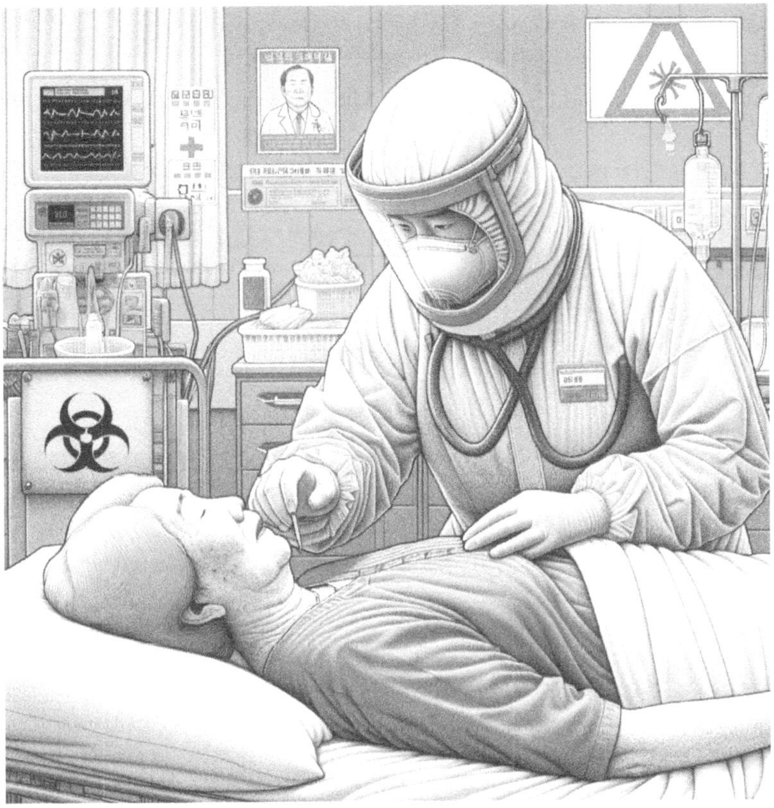

THE ORIGINS OF QUARANTINE: RAGUSA AND BEYOND

The Adriatic port city of Ragusa (modern-day Dubrovnik) played a pioneering role in the implementation of quarantine measures. In 1377, amid fears of the bubonic plague, Ragusa's Major Council passed a law requiring a mandatory quarantine period for those arriving from plague-infested areas. Individuals were required to spend a month on the islet of Mrkan or in the town of Cavtat for disinfection purposes. This practice evolved into a standard 40-day isolation period, deriving from the Latin "quadragina" and the Italian "quaranta," both meaning 40.

QUARANTINE IN ENGLAND

In the 16th Century, England adopted home quarantine measures to combat the plague. Houses with plague patients were marked with a red cross to prevent person-to-person transmission.

MODERN QUARANTINE AND ISOLATION

Quarantine today refers to restricting the movement of healthy individuals who may have been exposed to a contagious disease, while isolation involves separating and restricting the movement of sick individuals. These practices are usually implemented in homes, hospitals, or special facilities.

UNDERSTANDING OUTBREAKS, EPIDEMICS, AND PANDEMICS

The terms "outbreak," "epidemic," and "pandemic" describe the escalation of infectious diseases:

- An **outbreak** is a sudden increase in the number of disease cases.
- An **epidemic** affects many individuals at the same time in a specific area.
- A **pandemic** is an epidemic that spreads over a large area, potentially globally.

THE ROLE OF BIOSAFETY LEVELS

Biosafety levels (BSL) are set to contain infectious agents. They range from BSL-1, the lowest level, to BSL-4, the highest:

1. **Biosafety Level 1 (BSL-1)**: For non-human infectious agents. Standard laboratory practices are followed, and personal protective equipment (PPE) is minimal.
2. **Biosafety Level 2 (BSL-2)**: For moderate-risk agents. Access is limited, and specific training is required. Protective clothing, gloves, and eye protection are mandatory.
3. **Biosafety Level 3 (BSL-3)**: For diseases that can cause serious and potentially lethal infections. All work is performed in safety cabinets, and laboratory personnel must wear solid-front protective clothing.
4. **Biosafety Level 4 (BSL-4)**: For high-risk agents that pose a severe threat to individuals and public health. Facilities are either cabinet laboratories or protective-suit laboratories, designed to study deadly diseases like Ebola and Marburg viruses.

BSL-4 LABORATORIES IN EAST ASIA

Several countries in East Asia have established BSL-4 laboratories to research and manage highly infectious diseases:

- **China**: The Wuhan Institute of Virology (中国科学院武汉病毒研究所) in Wuhan, Hubei, became operational in 2015, hosting the first and only visible BSL-4 lab in China.
- **Japan**: The National Institute for Infectious Diseases (国立感染症研究所) in Tokyo and the Institute of Physical and Chemical Research (理化学研究所) in Tsukuba are key facilities.
- **South Korea**: The Korea Centers for Disease Control and Prevention (질병관리본부) in Cheongju opened its first BSL-4 lab in 2017.

- **Taiwan**: The Institute of Epidemiology and Preventive Medicine (流行病學與預防醫學研究所) at the National Defense University serves as a national university research center.

The history of quarantine and the development of biosafety measures reflect humanity's ongoing battle against infectious diseases. From the first quarantine in Ragusa to the modern network of high-level biosafety labs, these measures have been crucial in preventing the spread of diseases and protecting public health. Understanding these developments is key to appreciating the complexities and challenges of managing infectious diseases globally.

TASK 1: FILL IN THE BLANKS

1. In the 14th century, a prominent Adriatic port city was the first to implement mandatory __________ measures for incoming ships and caravans.
2. The term "quarantine" originates from the _______ and _______ words for the number 40.
3. During the 16th century in England, homes with plague patients were marked with a ______ cross to indicate quarantine.
4. __________ refers to the restriction of movement of healthy individuals who may have been exposed to a contagious disease.
5. __________ involves separating sick individuals with a contagious disease to prevent transmission to others.
6. An __________ is a sudden increase in the number of people infected with a disease.
7. An __________ affects many people at the same time in a specific area where the disease is not permanently prevalent.
8. A __________ is an epidemic that has spread over a large area, such as an entire country or continent.
9. Biosafety Level 1 (BSL-1) laboratories are generally used for diseases that do not infect __________.
10. At Biosafety Level 3 (BSL-3), laboratory personnel must wear __________ protective clothing.
11. Biosafety Level 4 (BSL-4) is the highest level of biosafety precautions, appropriate for work with agents that cause severe to fatal disease and for which there are no available __________ or __________.
12. The first person to become infected in an outbreak is often referred to as "__________ Zero."
13. BSL-4 laboratories are designed to handle deadly diseases, including several viruses known to cause viral __________ fever.

14. In BSL-4 labs, research may be conducted in cabinet laboratories or in __________-suit laboratories.

15. BSL-2 labs are suitable for work involving agents of moderate potential hazard to __________ and the __________.

TASK 2: LET'S TALK

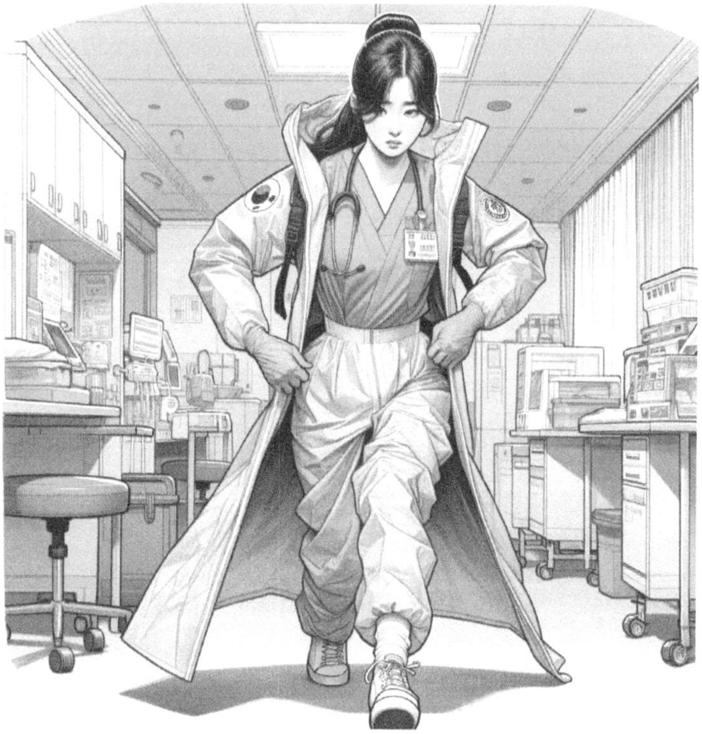

Nurse Alex (rushing in): Jordan, we've got an emergency! There's an outbreak of an unknown virus in the hospital. It's highly infectious!

Nurse Jordan: Oh no, that sounds serious. What do we need to do?

Nurse Alex: First, we need to get into hazmat suits immediately. They're in the BSL-4 storage room. We can't take any chances with this virus.

Nurse Jordan: Right, I'll head there now. Do we know how it's spreading?

Nurse Alex: Not yet, but we're treating it like a highly contagious airborne pathogen. We're setting up isolation units for the infected patients.

Nurse Jordan: I'll make sure to follow the BSL-4 protocols. What about the rest of the staff and patients?

Nurse Alex: The hospital is being locked down. No one in or out. We're also starting contact tracing to identify anyone who might have been exposed.

Nurse Jordan: Got it. What about protective measures for those who aren't in hazmat suits?

Nurse Alex: They should wear N95 masks at all times and follow strict hand hygiene protocols. We can't risk any further spread.

Nurse Jordan: Understood. Should we also prepare the antiviral medications, just in case?

Nurse Alex: Yes, get them ready. But remember, we don't know what we're dealing with yet. We'll need to wait for the virology team's analysis.

Nurse Jordan: I'm on it. Let's hope we can contain this quickly.

Nurse Alex: Agreed. Let's move fast and stay safe. I'll coordinate with the CDC and other health agencies. We need all the help we can get.

TASK 3: DO YOU REMEMBER?

1. **What type of protective suit do nurses need to wear during an outbreak of an unknown virus?**

____
____
____

2. **Where are the hazmat suits stored in a hospital during a viral outbreak?**

____
____
____

3. **What type of virus is causing the emergency in the hospital, according to the conversation?**

____
____
____

4. **What level of Biosafety protocols should be followed in the case of an aggressive virus outbreak?**

____
____
____

5. **How is the hospital responding to the outbreak of the unknown virus?**

6. **What measures are taken to prevent the spread of the virus within the hospital?**

7. **What is the protocol for staff and patient movement during the outbreak?**

8. **How does the hospital plan to identify individuals who might have been exposed to the virus?**

9. **What personal protective equipment should hospital staff wear if they are not in hazmat suits?**

10. **Are antiviral medications being prepared as a precaution, and what is the caution in using them?**

11. **Who is the hospital coordinating with for additional help and guidance during the outbreak?**

12. **What type of masks should be worn by those not in hazmat suits?**

13. **What is the presumed method of transmission of the unknown virus in the hospital?**

14. **What kind of units are being set up in the hospital for patients infected with the virus?**

15. **Why is there a need to wait for the virology team's analysis before administering treatment?**

TASK 4: LATIN AND GREEK TIME

1. **Quarantine**

    - Derived from the Latin "quadraginta" and the Italian "quaranta," both meaning 40, referring to the 40-day isolation period.

2. **Ragusa**

- Named after the Adriatic port city, not directly derived from Latin or Greek.

3. **Disinfection**

- *Dis-* comes from the Latin "dis," meaning apart, away.
- *Infection* comes from the Latin "infectio," meaning to dye, stain, or infect.

4. **Epidemic**

- Derived from the Greek words "epi" (ἐπί), meaning upon, and "demos" (δῆμος), meaning people.

5. **Pandemic**

- *Pan-* comes from the Greek "pan" (πᾶν), meaning all.
- *Demic* as in epidemic.

6. **Biosafety**

- *Bio-* comes from the Greek "bios" (βίος), meaning life.
- *Safety* comes from the Old French "sauf," meaning safe, not directly from Latin or Greek.

7. **Laboratories**

- Derived from the Latin "laboratorium," meaning a place to labor, work.

8. **Infectious**

- Comes from the Latin "infectiosus," meaning infectious or corrupting.

9. **Isolation**

- Derived from the Latin "insulatus," meaning made into an island.

10. **Agents**

- Comes from the Latin "agens," meaning doing, driving.

11. **Protective**

- Derived from the Latin "protectivus," meaning that which protects.

12. **Clothing**

- Comes from the Old English "clathung," not directly from Latin or Greek.

13. **Ebola**

- Named after the Ebola River in the Democratic Republic of Congo, not directly derived from Latin or Greek.

14. **Marburg**

- Named after the city of Marburg, Germany, not directly derived from Latin or Greek.

15. **Institute**

- Derived from the Latin "institutum," meaning something established or set up.

16. **Virology**

- *Virus* comes from the Latin "virus," meaning poison, venom.
- *-logy* as in biology.

17. **Epidemiology**

- *Epi-* and *-demos* as in epidemic.
- *-logy* as in biology.

18. **Preventive**

- Derived from the Latin "praeventivus," meaning going before or preceding

TASK 5: MAKE A CHOICE

1. The concept of quarantine was first implemented in:

A) Rome B) England

C) Ragusa (modern-day Dubrovnik) D) China

2. What was the original duration of the quarantine period in Ragusa?

A) 14 days B) 30 days C) 40 days D) 60 days

3. Quarantine in Ragusa was established in response to fears of:

A) Smallpox B) The bubonic plague

C) Influenza D) Cholera

4. In the 16th Century, what method did England adopt to combat the plague?

A) Vaccination B) Home quarantine

C) Building special hospitals D) Wearing protective suits

5. Modern quarantine refers to:

A) Isolating only sick individuals

B) Restricting movement of healthy individuals who may have been exposed

C) Mandatory vaccination

D) Complete lockdown of a city

6. What does an "outbreak" refer to?

A) A pandemic

B) A sudden increase in the number of disease cases

C) A long-term increase in disease cases

D) A global health crisis

7. Biosafety Level 1 (BSL-1) is suitable for:

A) High-risk agents like Ebola

B) Non-human infectious agents

C) Diseases causing serious infections

D) Research on common bacteria

8. What characterizes Biosafety Level 2 (BSL-2)?

A) Minimal protective measures

B) Research on moderate-risk agents

C) Use of cabinet laboratories

D) Study of non-infectious materials

9. Which level of biosafety involves working in safety cabinets for serious infections?

A) BSL-1 B) BSL-2 C) BSL-3 D) BSL-4

10. Biosafety Level 4 (BSL-4) laboratories are designed for:

A) Low-risk microbiological studies

B) High-risk agents posing severe threats

C) Basic scientific research

D) Educational purposes

11. The first BSL-4 lab in China was established in:

A) Beijing B) Shanghai C) Wuhan D) Guangzhou

12. The National Institute for Infectious Diseases in Japan is an example of a:

A) BSL-2 facility B) BSL-3 facility

C) BSL-4 facility D) General medical laboratory

13. What is the primary purpose of quarantine?

A) Research on new medicines

B) Preventing the spread of diseases

C) Psychological assessment

D) Physical training

14. Lymphedema in the context of biosafety refers to:

A) A type of cancer

B) Swelling due to lymph accumulation

C) A respiratory condition

D) A skin infection

15. Isolation differs from quarantine in that it involves:

A) Separating and restricting movement of healthy individuals

B) Separating and restricting movement of sick individuals

C) Global travel restrictions

D) Mandatory vaccinations

Chapter 15: Childhood Development

Childhood development is a complex and multifaceted process. Two of the most influential theorists in this field are Jean Piaget and Lev Vygotsky. Their theories, though different in approaches, offer profound insights into how children grow, learn, and understand the world around them.

JEAN PIAGET: STAGES OF COGNITIVE DEVELOPMENT

BACKGROUND

Jean Piaget, a Swiss psychologist born in 1896, was a pioneering figure in the study of child development. His theory of cognitive development is a comprehensive model of the inner workings of the young mind.

KEY CONCEPTS

Piaget's theory is structured around the idea that children progress through a series of four distinct stages of cognitive development:

1. **Sensorimotor Stage (Birth to 2 Years)**: In this stage, infants learn through interacting with their environment using their senses and motor skills. Key developments include the understanding of object permanence and the realization of self as a separate entity from the environment.

2. **Preoperational Stage (2 to 7 Years)**: Children begin to use language and think symbolically, yet their thinking is still intuitive and egocentric. They struggle to see things from perspectives other than their own.

3. **Concrete Operational Stage (7 to 11 Years)**: During this phase, children start thinking logically about concrete events. They understand the concept of conservation – that quantity remains the same despite changes in shape or arrangement.

4. **Formal Operational Stage (12 Years and Up)**: Adolescents develop the ability to think about abstract concepts. They can reason hypothetically and consider future possibilities.

Piaget's theory emphasizes that children actively construct their understanding of the world through their experiences and interactions.

LEV VYGOTSKY: SOCIOCULTURAL THEORY OF COGNITIVE DEVELOPMENT

BACKGROUND

Lev Vygotsky, born in Russia in 1896, provided a stark contrast to Piaget with his sociocultural theory of cognitive development. He focused on the roles of social interaction and cultural context in shaping a child's cognitive development.

KEY CONCEPTS

Vygotsky's theory is based on three fundamental principles:

1. **Social Interaction Influences Cognitive Development**: Vygotsky believed that learning is a social process. Through interactions with more knowledgeable others (parents, teachers, peers), children learn new skills and acquire new knowledge.
2. **The Zone of Proximal Development (ZPD)**: This concept refers to the difference between what a child can achieve independently and what they can achieve with guidance and encouragement from a skilled partner. The ZPD represents the potential for cognitive development.
3. **Language and Thought**: Vygotsky considered language as a critical tool of cognitive development. For him, internal speech was particularly important as a means of thinking and problem-solving.

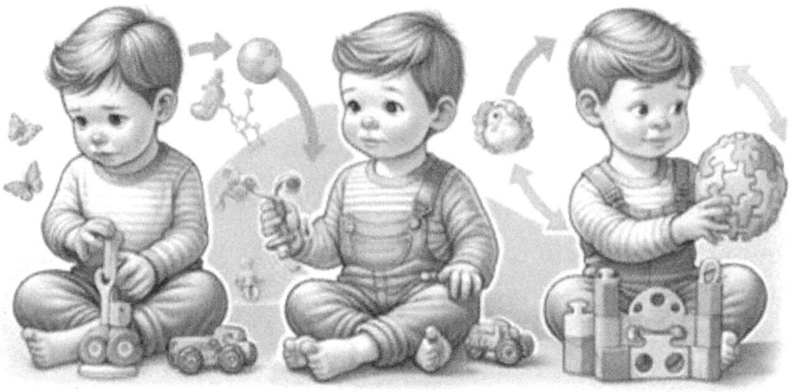

COMPARING AND CONTRASTING PIAGET AND VYGOTSKY

While Piaget emphasized stages of development and intrinsic cognitive maturation, Vygotsky focused on the external influences of culture and social interaction. Piaget saw children as solitary explorers of their world, whereas Vygotsky viewed them as social learners, deeply influenced by their cultural context.

APPLICATION IN EDUCATION

In education, Piaget's theory underscores the importance of age-appropriate learning and the stages of cognitive readiness. Vygotsky's theory, on the other hand, highlights the importance of teacher-student interaction, peer collaboration, and the role of language in learning.

TASK 1: FILL IN THE BLANKS

1. Jean _______ and Lev _______ are influential theorists in the field of _______ development.
2. Piaget's theory is structured around _______ stages of cognitive development.

3. In the _______ stage, infants learn through senses and motor skills, developing an understanding of _______ permanence.

4. The _______ Operational Stage is when children start thinking logically about concrete events and understand the concept of _______.

5. Vygotsky's theory emphasizes that cognitive development is shaped by _______ interaction and _______ context.

6. The _______ of Proximal Development is a concept by Vygotsky, highlighting the potential for cognitive development through _______ guidance.

7. According to Vygotsky, _______ is a critical tool in cognitive development, especially internal _______.

8. Piaget viewed children as _______ explorers, while Vygotsky saw them as _______ learners.

9. In education, Piaget's theory underscores the importance of age-appropriate _______ and cognitive _______.

10. Vygotsky's approach in education focuses on the role of _______-student interaction and the importance of _______ in learning.

TASK 2: LET'S TALK

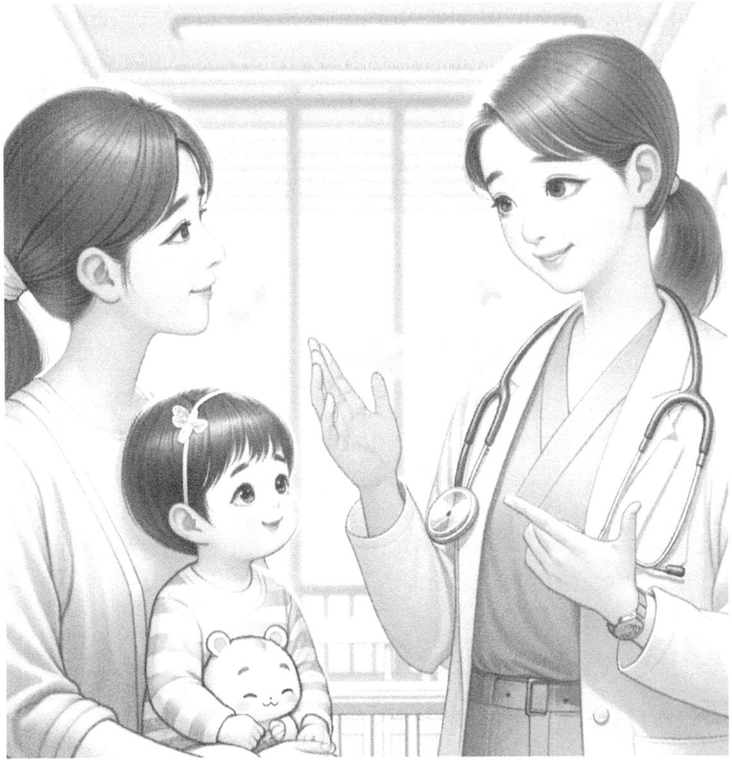

Emma: Hello Rachel, how are you and little Sophie doing today?

Rachel: Hi Emma, we're doing well. I'm just a bit anxious about Sophie's development. She's almost two now, and I want to make sure she's on track.

Emma: That's perfectly normal. At her age, children are in what Jean Piaget called the Sensorimotor Stage of development. It's a time when they explore the world through their senses and actions.

Rachel: Yes, she's very curious, always touching and tasting things!

Emma: That's exactly what she should be doing. It's how children learn at this stage. They also start understanding object permanence – realizing that things still exist even when they can't see them.

Rachel: I've noticed that with her toys. She looks for them even when they're hidden. Is there anything else I should encourage?

Emma: It's great to engage her in different activities that stimulate her senses. Simple games like 'peek-a-boo' are actually beneficial. As she grows, she'll enter what Piaget termed the Preoperational Stage, where language and symbolic play become important.

Rachel: What about social development? I want her to start playing well with others.

Emma: Social interaction is essential, as Lev Vygotsky emphasized. He believed that children learn a lot through interactions. Playdates and group activities are great for this.

Rachel: I've been reading to her and talking to her a lot. Does that help?

Emma: Absolutely. Language development is crucial. Vygotsky stated that language is a key tool in cognitive development. Reading and talking to her will greatly aid her learning and understanding of the world.

Rachel: What can I do to help her in her next stages of development?

Emma: Continue being interactive. As she grows, focus on activities that challenge her thinking but are still within her capabilities – what Vygotsky called the Zone of Proximal Development. It's about helping her learn with a little guidance, but not doing everything for her.

Rachel: That makes sense. I want to support her learning as best as I can.

Emma: You're doing a great job. Remember, every child develops at their own pace, and these stages are just guidelines. If you have any concerns, we're here to help.

Rachel: Thank you, Emma. This information really helps me understand what Sophie is going through and how I can support her.

TASK 3: DO YOU REMEMBER?

1. **Who are the two influential theorists mentioned in the article on childhood development?**

2. **What is the name of the first stage of cognitive development according to Piaget?**

3. **During the Sensorimotor Stage, children develop an understanding of what key concept?**

4. **What kind of play becomes important in Piaget's Preoperational Stage?**

5. **According to Vygotsky, what plays a crucial role in a child's cognitive development?**

6. **What did Vygotsky call the difference between what a child can do alone and with help?**

7. **How does Vygotsky describe the role of language in cognitive development?**

8. **What did the nurse suggest as beneficial activities for a two-year-old child?**

9. **Why are playdates and group activities important for a child, as per Vygotsky's theory?**

10. **What is an example of a simple game beneficial for children in the Sensorimotor Stage?**

11. **How can parents support their child's learning in the Zone of Proximal Development?**

12. **What did the nurse advise about reading and talking to the child?**

13. **What did the nurse advise about reading and talking to the child?**

14. **What advice did the nurse give regarding the pace of a child's development?**

TASK 4: LATIN AND GREEK TIME

1. **Sensorimotor**

- *Sensori-* comes from the Latin word "sensus," meaning sense.
- *Motor* comes from the Latin word "motor," meaning mover.

2. **Preoperational**

- *Pre-* comes from the Latin word "prae," meaning before.
- *Operational* comes from the Latin word "operatio," meaning work, labor, or operation.

3. **Concrete**

- Derived from the Latin word "concretus," meaning grown together, hardened.

4. **Formal**

- Comes from the Latin word "formalis," meaning pertaining to form.

5. **Sociocultural**

- *Socio-* comes from the Latin word "socius," meaning companion, ally.
- *Cultural* comes from the Latin word "cultura," meaning cultivation or culture.

6. **Interaction**

- *Inter-* comes from the Latin word "inter," meaning between.
- *Action* comes from the Latin word "actio," meaning a doing, a driving.

7. **Zone of Proximal Development (ZPD)**

- *Zone* comes from the Greek word "zōnē" (ζώνη), meaning belt or girdle.
- *Proximal* comes from the Latin word "proximus," meaning nearest.
- *Development* as above.

8. **Language**

- Derived from the Latin word "lingua," meaning tongue or language.

9. **Contrasting**

- Comes from the Latin word "contra," meaning against, and "stare," meaning to stand.

10. **Education**

- Derived from the Latin word "educatio," meaning a breeding, a bringing up, a rearing.

11. **Interaction**

- *Inter-* as above.
- *Action* as above.

12. **Collaboration**

- Comes from the Latin word "collaborare," meaning to work together.

TASK 5: MAKE A CHOICE

1. Jean Piaget is best known for his work in:

A) Sociocultural development B) Cognitive development

C) Behavioral psychology D) Psychoanalysis

2. Piaget's theory of cognitive development includes how many distinct stages?

A) Two B) Three C) Four D) Five

3. The Sensorimotor Stage, according to Piaget, occurs from:

A) Birth to 2 years B) 2 to 7 years

C) 7 to 11 years D) 12 years and up

4. In Piaget's theory, the understanding of object permanence develops in which stage?

A) Sensorimotor Stage B) Preoperational Stage

C) Concrete Operational Stage D) Formal Operational Stage

5. Lev Vygotsky's theory emphasizes the role of what in cognitive development?

A) Individual exploration B) Biological factors

C) Social interaction D) Fixed stages of development

6. Vygotsky introduced the concept of:

A) Conservation B) Object permanence

C) Zone of Proximal Development D) Abstract reasoning

7. Which theorist focused on the stages of cognitive readiness in education?

A) Piaget B) Vygotsky C) Freud D) Skinner

8. Vygotsky's theory highlights the importance of what in learning?

A) Peer collaboration B) Strict curriculums

C) Solitary learning D) Punishment and rewards

9. According to Piaget, egocentric thinking is most characteristic of which stage?

A) Sensorimotor Stage

B) Preoperational Stage

C) Concrete Operational Stage

D) Formal Operational Stage

10. Who proposed that language is crucial for cognitive development?

A) Piaget B) Vygotsky C) Erikson D) Bandura

11. The ability to think logically about concrete events is part of Piaget's:

A) Sensorimotor Stage

B) Preoperational Stage

C) Concrete Operational Stage

D) Formal Operational Stage

12. The concept of internal speech was emphasized by:

A) Piaget B) Vygotsky C) Kohlberg D) Ainsworth

13. According to Piaget, at what stage can a child reason hypothetically?

A) Sensorimotor Stage

B) Preoperational Stage

C) Concrete Operational Stage

D) Formal Operational Stage

14. Vygotsky believed that learning is:

A) A biological process B) A social process

C) A solitary process D) An unchangeable process

15. Piaget's theory suggests that children:

A) Rely on adults for learning

B) Construct understanding through experiences

C) Learn best in group settings

D) Have little role in their cognitive development

Chapter 16: Paediatric Disease

Childhood is often accompanied by a series of common illnesses that, while usually mild, require proper care and attention. Among these, measles, chickenpox, rubella, jaundice, and diaper rash are notable for their prevalence and impact. This article discusses the symptoms and treatment of these conditions, aiming to provide parents and caregivers with essential information for effective management.

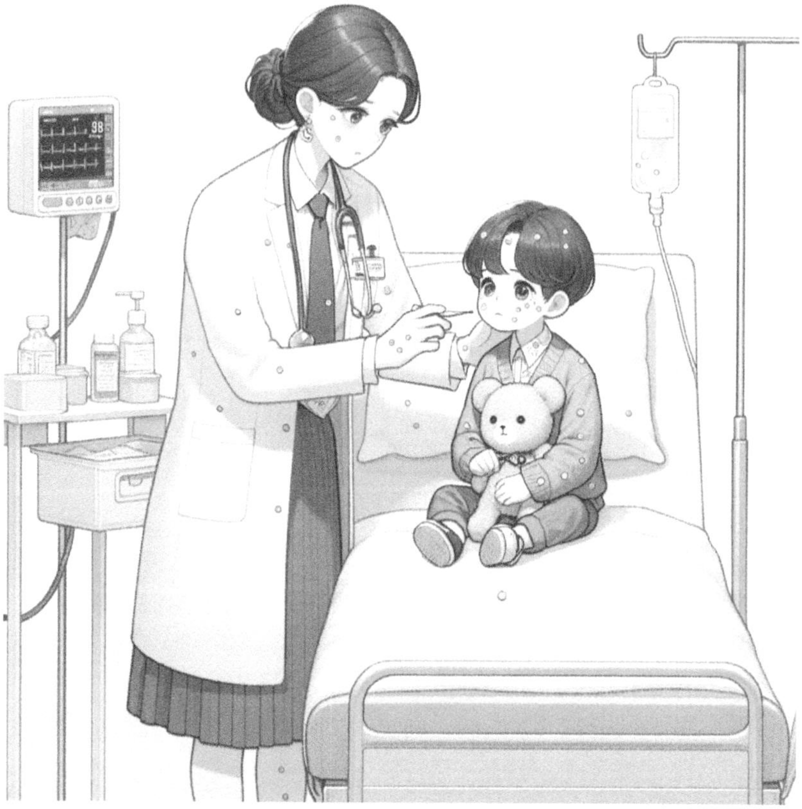

Measles

- **Symptoms:** High fever, cough, runny nose, red, watery eyes, followed by a rash that spreads over the body.
- **Treatment:** No specific antiviral treatment; care is supportive. This includes bed rest, hydration, and fever management with acetaminophen or ibuprofen. Vitamin A supplements may be recommended.
- **Prevention:** Vaccination with the MMR (measles, mumps, rubella) vaccine is the most effective preventive measure.

Chickenpox (Varicella)

- **Symptoms:** Fever, tiredness, loss of appetite, followed by a characteristic itchy rash that forms blisters and scabs.
- **Treatment:** Calamine lotion and oatmeal baths can help relieve itching. Paracetamol can be used for fever. Antiviral medication may be prescribed in severe cases.
- **Prevention:** The varicella vaccine is effective in preventing chickenpox and is part of routine childhood immunization schedules.

Rubella (German Measles)

- **Symptoms:** Low-grade fever, sore throat, rash that starts on the face and spreads to the rest of the body, swollen lymph nodes.
- **Treatment:** Like measles, treatment is mainly supportive, focusing on relieving symptoms. There is no specific antiviral treatment.
- **Prevention:** Vaccination with the MMR vaccine is key to preventing rubella.

Jaundice in Newborns

- **Symptoms:** Yellowing of the skin and the whites of the eyes, poor feeding, lethargy.
- **Treatment:** Mild jaundice often disappears on its own. More severe cases may require phototherapy (light therapy).
- **Management:** Regular monitoring of jaundice levels, ensuring the baby is feeding well, and routine check-ups are important.

Diaper Rash

- **Symptoms:** Red, inflamed skin in the diaper area.
- **Treatment:** Keeping the area clean and dry is crucial. Changing diapers frequently, using water-based wipes or water for cleaning, and applying barrier creams can help. In cases of a yeast infection, antifungal creams may be prescribed.
- **Prevention:** Regular diaper changes, good hygiene, and airing out the skin can help prevent diaper rash.

While common, these childhood illnesses each have unique symptoms and treatment approaches. Understanding these can greatly assist in providing appropriate care and comfort to the child. Vaccinations play a critical role in preventing many of these diseases, highlighting the importance of adhering to recommended immunization schedules. In all cases, if there is any concern about the severity of symptoms or the effectiveness of home-based treatments, seeking medical advice is essential. Early intervention and proper management are key to ensuring the health and well-being of children during these illnesses.

TASK 1: FILL IN THE BLANKS

1. Measles is characterized by a high fever, cough, runny nose, and a rash that spreads over the body. Treatment is mainly __________.

2. Chickenpox, also known as __________, causes an itchy rash with blisters and can be prevented through __________.

3. __________, also known as German measles, presents with symptoms like a low-grade fever and a rash starting on the face.

4. Newborn jaundice results in the yellowing of the skin and eyes, and severe cases may require __________ for treatment.

5. Diaper rash causes red, inflamed skin in the diaper area and is treated by keeping the area __________ and __________.

6. To relieve the symptoms of measles, __________ supplements may be recommended alongside supportive care.

7. The varicella vaccine is used to prevent __________ in children as part of routine immunizations.

8. The MMR vaccine protects against measles, mumps, and __________.

9. Phototherapy, a treatment involving __________, is often used to treat severe cases of __________ in newborns.

10. For diaper rash, changing diapers __________ and using __________ creams can help prevent and treat the condition.

TASK 2: LET'S TALK

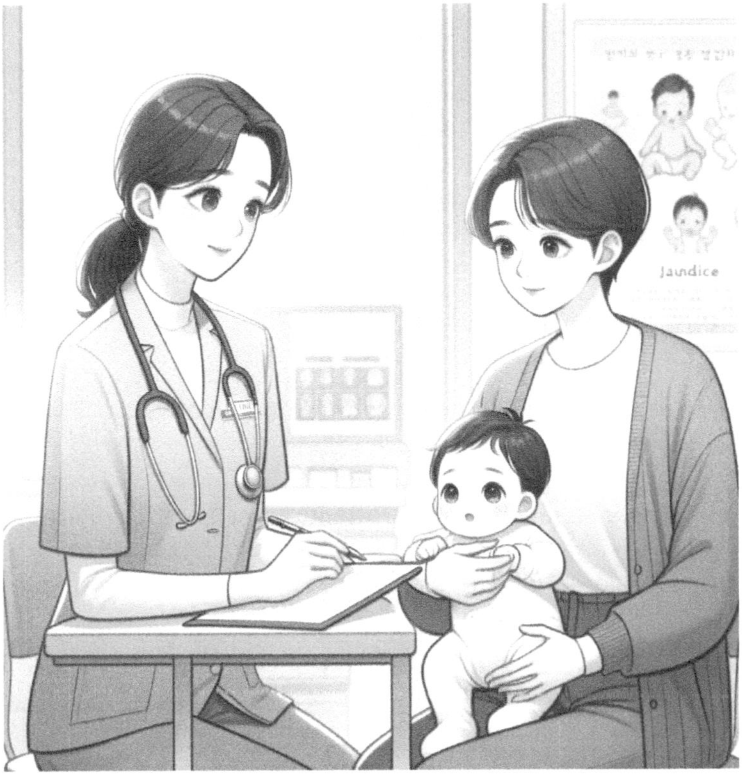

Mother: Yes, thank you. I'm a bit worried. I noticed his skin and eyes are a bit yellow. Why does this happen?

Nurse: That's a great question. Newborn jaundice is quite common and usually not a cause for alarm. It happens due to bilirubin, which is a byproduct of the normal breakdown of red blood cells. In adults and older children, the liver processes bilirubin, which is then excreted. However, in newborns, the liver is often not mature enough to get rid of bilirubin effectively, leading to a build-up and causing the skin and eyes to appear yellow.

Mother: Is it dangerous? What should we do?

Nurse: In most cases, it's a temporary condition and resolves on its own as the baby's liver matures. However, we monitor it closely because if the bilirubin level becomes too high, it could be harmful. That's where the treatment comes in – we use what's called 'bili lights' or phototherapy.

Mother: Phototherapy? How does that work?

Nurse: It's quite fascinating, actually. Phototherapy involves placing your baby under a type of light that emits blue spectrum light. This light alters the bilirubin in your baby's body, turning it into a form that can be excreted more easily through urine and stool. It's a safe and effective way to lower bilirubin levels.

Mother: Will my baby be comfortable during this treatment?

Nurse: Absolutely. Your baby will be in a warm, secure incubator and will wear protective eyewear to rest comfortably under the lights. We ensure they are well cared for and monitored throughout the treatment.

Mother: How long does the treatment usually take?

Nurse: It varies depending on the bilirubin levels and how the baby responds to the treatment. Some babies need only a day or two, while others might need a bit longer. We'll be checking the bilirubin levels regularly to determine how long the treatment should continue.

Mother: Is there anything I can do to help?

Nurse: Yes, feeding your baby frequently helps. The more they feed, the more they'll urinate and pass stools, which helps eliminate bilirubin from their system. And of course, we're here for any questions or assistance you need.

Mother: Thank you so much. This information really eases my mind.

Nurse: You're welcome! It's important to us that you feel informed and comfortable with your baby's care. We're here every step of the way.

TASK 3: DO YOU REMEMBER?

1. **What is the common term for Varicella?**

____

____

____

2. **Which vaccine is used to prevent Chickenpox?**

____

____

____

3. **What are the main symptoms of Rubella, also known as German Measles?**

____

____

____

4. **What is the primary cause of newborn jaundice?**

5. **How does phototherapy help in treating newborn jaundice?**

6. **What color is the light used in phototherapy for jaundice treatment?**

7. **Why are newborns more susceptible to jaundice compared to adults?**

8. **What symptom is common to both measles and rubella in children?**

9. **How is diaper rash typically treated?**

10. **Which organ in newborns is often not mature enough to effectively process bilirubin?**

11. **In the conversation, what does the nurse recommend to help reduce bilirubin levels, besides phototherapy?**

12. **What type of protective gear is used for babies during phototherapy?**

13. **What is the main treatment for measles in children?**

14. **How can Chickenpox be prevented, besides vaccination?**

15. **According to the article, what is a common symptom of Chickenpox?**

TASK 4: LATIN AND GREEK TIME

1. **Measles**

- The term "measles" does not have a clear Latin or Greek origin. It is derived from the Middle Dutch word "masel," meaning blemish.

2. **Symptoms**

- Derived from the Greek word "symptoma" (σύμπτωμα), meaning a happening, accident, disease.

3. **Treatment**

- Comes from the Latin word "tractare," meaning to handle, manage, deal with.

4. **Prevention**

- Derived from the Latin word "praeventionem," meaning action of hindering.

5. **Vaccination**

- Comes from the Latin word "vacca," meaning cow, a reference to cowpox virus used in early vaccinations.

6. **Chickenpox (Varicella)**

- *Chickenpox* does not have a clear Latin or Greek origin. It's possibly derived from chickpeas (due to the blisters' resemblance) or from the Old English "gican," meaning to itch.
- *Varicella* comes from the Latin word "varius," meaning spotted.

7. **Rubella (German Measles)**

- *Rubella* is derived from the Latin word "rubellus," meaning little red.
- *German Measles* is a colloquial name, not derived from Latin or Greek.

8. **Jaundice**

- Comes from the French word "jaunisse," meaning yellowness, from "jaune," yellow.

9. **Phototherapy**

- *Photo-* comes from the Greek word "phos" (φῶς), meaning light.
- *-therapy* comes from the Greek word "therapeia" (θεραπεία), meaning healing, curing.

10. **Diaper Rash**

- *Diaper* comes from the Greek word "diapēra," meaning a cloth, towel.

- *Rash* comes from the Middle English "rasch," not directly from Latin or Greek.

11. **Inflammation**

- Derived from the Latin word "inflammare," meaning to set on fire.

12. **Hygiene**

- Comes from the Greek word "hygieine" (ὑγιεινή), pertaining to health, from "Hygieia," the Greek goddess of health.

13. **Immunization**

- Derived from the Latin word "immunis," meaning exempt, free.

14. **Paracetamol**

- The name is derived from its chemical name: para-acetylaminophenol.

15. **Antifungal**

- *Anti-* comes from the Greek word "anti" (ἀντί), meaning against.
- *Fungal* comes from the Latin word "fungus," meaning mushroom, fungus.

TASK 5: MAKE A CHOICE

1. What is a common symptom of measles?

A) Rash that spreads over the body

B) Yellowing of the skin

C) Persistent cough

D) Loss of appetite

2. Which is NOT a treatment for measles?

A) Specific antiviral treatment B) Hydration

C) Bed rest D) Fever management with acetaminophen

3. The most effective preventive measure for measles is:

A) Regular hand washing

B) Quarantine

C) Vaccination with the MMR vaccine

D) Use of antibacterial soap

4. Chickenpox symptoms include:

A) High fever and a characteristic itchy rash

B) Cough and runny nose

C) Sore throat and swollen lymph nodes

D) Red, inflamed skin in the diaper area

5. Treatment for chickenpox usually involves:

A) Phototherapy

B) Calamine lotion and oatmeal baths

C) Blood transfusion

D) High doses of antibiotics

6. Rubella, also known as German measles, typically features:

A) A low-grade fever and sore throat

B) Intense abdominal pain

C) Severe respiratory distress

D) Blister-like skin lesions

7. The primary symptom of jaundice in newborns is:

A) Yellowing of the skin and the whites of the eyes

B) A rash that spreads over the body

C) Severe itching and redness

D) High fever and cough

8. Severe cases of newborn jaundice may require:

A) Oatmeal baths B) Phototherapy

C) Vaccination D) Antibiotics

9. Diaper rash is characterized by:

A) High fever and cough

B) Red, inflamed skin in the diaper area

C) Yellowing of the skin

D) Loss of appetite and lethargy

10. A key prevention method for diaper rash is:

A) Regular diaper changes and good hygiene

B) Phototherapy

C) Antiviral medication

D) High doses of vitamin A

11. Which is a recommended treatment for diaper rash?

A) Calamine lotion

B) Antifungal creams for yeast infections

C) Acetaminophen or ibuprofen

D) High fluid intake

12. Which is NOT a symptom of chickenpox?

A) Loss of appetite B) Itchy rash forming blisters

C) Yellowing of the skin D) Fever and tiredness

13. Measles is preventable through:

A) High fluid intake B) Phototherapy

C) MMR vaccination D) Antibiotic treatment

14. What is the main focus of treatment for measles?

A) Specific antiviral medication B) Supportive care

C) Immediate vaccination D) Surgical intervention

15. Rubella is prevented primarily by:

A) The varicella vaccine

B) The MMR vaccine

C) Regular hand washing

D) Isolation of the infected individual

Chapter 17: Geriatric Diseases

The field of geriatric medicine focuses on health conditions that predominantly affect older adults. As we age, our bodies become more vulnerable to certain diseases, making the understanding and management of these conditions crucial for maintaining quality of life in the elderly. This article delves into some common geriatric diseases and discusses effective strategies for their management.

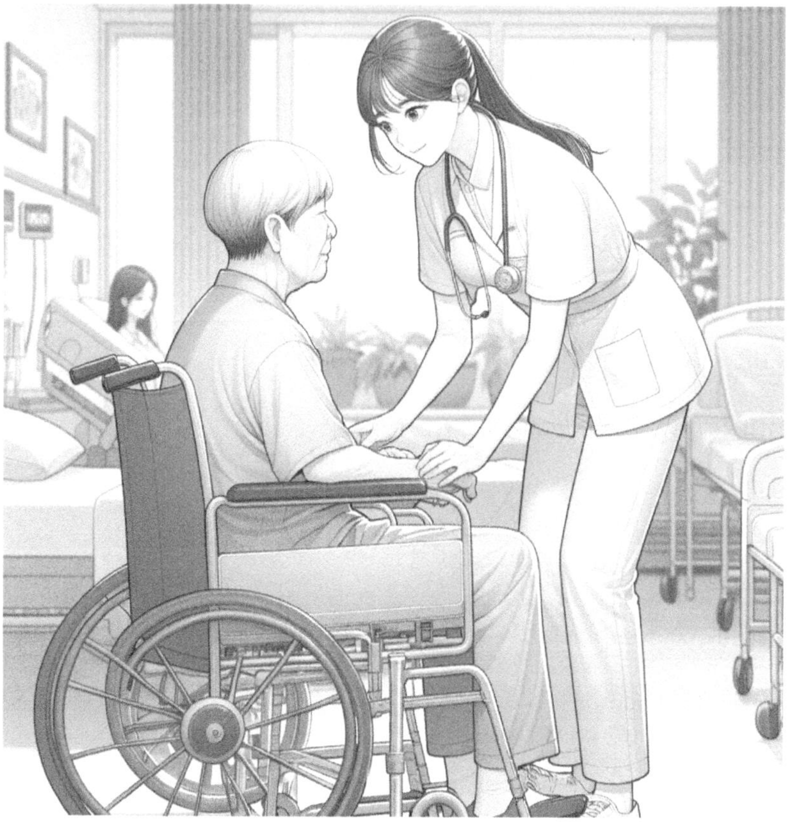

Cardiovascular Diseases in the Elderly

Cardiovascular diseases, such as hypertension, heart disease, and stroke, are prevalent in older adults. These conditions often manifest as shortness of breath, chest pain, and dizziness. Management typically involves lifestyle modifications, including a healthy diet and regular exercise. Medications to control blood pressure and cholesterol levels are also commonly prescribed, along with regular cardiovascular health check-ups to monitor and manage these conditions effectively.

The Challenge of Arthritis

Arthritis, including osteoarthritis and rheumatoid arthritis, is a significant concern for the elderly, characterized by joint pain, stiffness, and swelling. Management strategies encompass a combination of physical therapy, pain relief medications, and, in some cases, surgical interventions. Additionally, weight management and low-impact exercises can alleviate symptoms and improve joint function.

Battling Osteoporosis

Osteoporosis often remains undetected until a fracture occurs, making it a silent threat to many older adults. The management of osteoporosis includes the use of calcium and vitamin D supplements and medications that help strengthen the bones. Incorporating lifestyle changes, such as engaging in weight-bearing exercises, is also essential to improve bone density and reduce the risk of fractures.

Navigating Alzheimer's Disease and Dementia

Memory loss, confusion, and difficulty with communication and understanding are hallmark symptoms of Alzheimer's Disease and other forms of dementia. Managing these conditions involves medications to manage symptoms, cognitive therapy, and creating a safe and supportive living environment. Support for caregivers is also a critical component, as they play a vital role in the daily care of individuals with dementia.

Managing Diabetes in Older Adults

Diabetes is characterized by increased thirst, frequent urination, fatigue, and blurred vision. Effective management includes regular monitoring of blood sugar levels, adherence to a diabetic diet, regular exercise, and medications or insulin therapy, depending on the severity of the condition.

Addressing Chronic Obstructive Pulmonary Disease (COPD)

COPD is a chronic lung condition marked by a persistent cough, shortness of breath, and wheezing. Management strategies include smoking cessation, pulmonary rehabilitation, and medications like bronchodilators. In severe cases, oxygen therapy may be necessary.

Confronting Geriatric Depression

Depression in the elderly is often characterized by persistent sadness, loss of interest in activities, and changes in sleep and appetite. Management typically involves psychotherapy, antidepressant medications, and lifestyle interventions like regular physical activity and social engagement to improve overall mood and well-being.

Tackling Urinary Incontinence

Urinary incontinence, the loss of bladder control, can be a distressing condition for many older adults. Management includes pelvic floor exercises, bladder training, medications, and sometimes surgery. The use of absorbent pads and protective garments can also provide comfort and dignity.

Coping with Age-Related Macular Degeneration (AMD)

AMD affects central vision, making it difficult to recognize faces or perceive colors accurately. Management often involves dietary supplements and medications to slow the disease's progression. Using visual aids like magnifying glasses can also help those affected continue to engage in reading and other activities.

Dealing with Hearing Loss

Hearing loss in the elderly may manifest as difficulty in hearing conversations, especially in noisy environments. Management includes the use of hearing aids, cochlear implants in severe cases, and employing communication strategies such as lip-reading and sign language.

The management of geriatric diseases is a multifaceted approach that encompasses medical interventions, lifestyle adjustments, and supportive care. Early detection and regular monitoring play a crucial role in the effective management of these conditions. The involvement of caregivers and family members is also vital, providing necessary support and adjustments to improve the elderly's quality of life. With advancements in medical science, new and improved treatments continue to emerge, offering better care and hope for the elderly population.

TASK 1: FILL IN THE BLANKS

1. Cardiovascular diseases in older adults often manifest as __________.

2. Lifestyle modifications for managing cardiovascular diseases include a healthy __________ and regular __________.

3. __________, including osteoarthritis and rheumatoid arthritis, causes joint pain and stiffness in the elderly.

4. The management of arthritis might involve __________ therapy and pain relief __________.

5. __________ often remains asymptomatic in the elderly until a fracture occurs.

6. Alzheimer's Disease and other forms of dementia are characterized by __________ loss, confusion, and difficulty with communication.

7. Managing diabetes in older adults involves monitoring __________ levels and adhering to a diabetic __________.

8. COPD, a chronic lung condition, is marked by a persistent __________, shortness of breath, and wheezing.

9. Geriatric depression is often managed through __________, antidepressant medications, and lifestyle __________.

10. Urinary __________ in the elderly can be managed with pelvic floor exercises and __________ training.

11. Age-Related Macular Degeneration (AMD) primarily affects __________ vision in older adults.

12. Management of AMD often involves dietary __________ and sometimes __________ to slow progression.

13. Hearing loss in the elderly may require the use of __________ aids or cochlear __________ in severe cases.

14. Osteoporosis management includes taking calcium and __________ D supplements.

15. For joint pain in arthritis, weight management and __________-impact exercises can be beneficial.

TASK 2: LET'S TALK

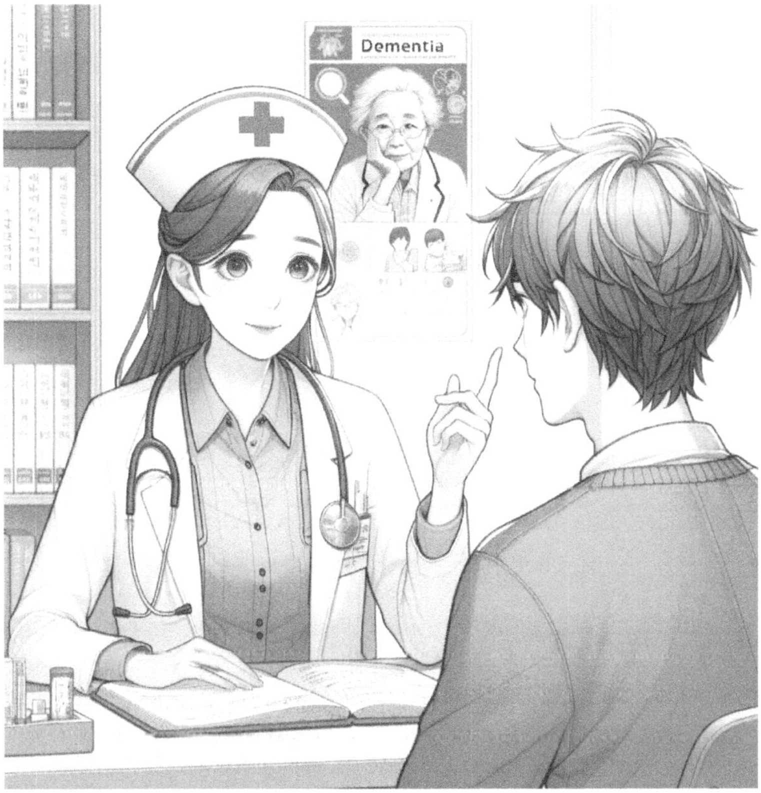

Nurse: Good afternoon, I'm Nurse Williams. I understand you're concerned about your father's recent changes in behavior and memory?

Adult Child 1 (Anna): Yes, Nurse Williams. We've noticed he's becoming more forgetful and sometimes he seems confused. It's not like him.

Adult Child 2 (Michael): He's been misplacing things and forgetting important dates, which he never used to do. We're really worried it might be Alzheimer's.

Nurse: It's good that you've noticed these changes. Alzheimer's is a common condition in the elderly, characterized by memory loss, confusion, and difficulty with communication. It's important to have a formal evaluation to confirm the diagnosis and understand the stage of the disease.

Anna: Is there a treatment that can help him?

Nurse: While there's no cure for Alzheimer's, there are medications that can help manage the symptoms. Cognitive therapy can also be beneficial. The key is creating a safe and supportive environment for him.

Michael: What can we do to make things easier for him at home?

Nurse: Simplifying his daily routine can reduce confusion. It's also helpful to use reminders, like notes or alarms, for important tasks or medications. Keeping the home environment calm and familiar is important.

Anna: What about his long-term care? Should we consider a nursing home?

Nurse: That decision depends on several factors, including the progression of his condition and your ability to care for him at home. Many families find that a combination of home care and professional support works well in the early stages. As the disease progresses, more intensive care may be needed.

Michael: How do we prepare for what's coming? It's all so overwhelming.

Nurse: It's a journey, and preparation is key. I recommend joining a support group for families dealing with Alzheimer's. They can provide valuable advice and emotional support. Also, it's important to keep regular medical check-ups for your father to monitor the progression of the disease.

Anna: Are there any lifestyle changes or activities that can help him?

Nurse: Absolutely. Regular physical activity, social interaction, and mentally stimulating activities can be beneficial. Also, ensure he has a balanced diet and stays hydrated.

Michael: Thank you, Nurse Williams. This information is really helpful.

Nurse: You're welcome. Remember, you're not alone in this. We're here to support you and your father through this journey. Don't hesitate to reach out if you have any more questions or need assistance.

TASK 3: DO YOU REMEMBER?

1. **What are common symptoms of Alzheimer's disease in the elderly?**

____

____

____

2. **What type of therapy can be beneficial for managing Alzheimer's symptoms?**

____

____

____

3. **In Alzheimer's management, why is creating a safe and supportive environment important?**

4. **What lifestyle modifications can help manage cardiovascular diseases in older adults?**

5. **What are two common types of arthritis that affect the elderly?**

6. **How can physical therapy help in the management of arthritis?**

7. **What silent condition in the elderly often remains undetected until a fracture occurs?**

8. **What dietary supplements are recommended for osteoporosis management?**

9. **Which chronic lung condition is marked by a persistent cough and shortness of breath in the elderly?**

10. **What management strategies are suggested for geriatric depression?**

11. **What condition in the elderly is characterized by the loss of bladder control?**

12. **How is Age-Related Macular Degeneration (AMD) typically managed?**

13. **What aids might be required for elderly individuals experiencing hearing loss?**

14. **In the conversation, what did the nurse suggest for simplifying the daily routine of an Alzheimer's patient?**

15. **What did the nurse recommend for the family to prepare for the progression of Alzheimer's disease?**

____

____

____

TASK 4: LATIN AND GREEK TIME

1. **Cardiovascular**

- *Cardio* comes from the Greek word "kardia" (καρδιά), meaning heart.
- *Vascular* comes from the Latin word "vasculum," meaning little vessel.

2. **Arthritis**

- *Arthr* comes from the Greek word "arthron" (ἄρθρον), meaning joint.
- *Itis* comes from the Greek word "itis" (ἴτις), meaning inflammation.

3. **Osteoporosis**

- *Osteo* comes from the Greek word "osteon" (ὀστέον), meaning bone.
- *Porosis* comes from the Greek word "poros" (πόρος), meaning pore or passage.

4. **Alzheimer's**

- Named after Alois Alzheimer, a German psychiatrist and neuropathologist. It does not have Latin or Greek roots.

5. **Dementia**

- Comes from the Latin word "demens," meaning out of one's mind.

6. **Diabetes**

- Comes from the Greek word "diabētēs" (διαβήτης), which refers to a siphon, to pass through.

7. **Pulmonary**

- Comes from the Latin word "pulmonarius," meaning of the lungs.

8. **Depression**

- Comes from the Latin word "deprimere," meaning to press down.

9. **Incontinence**

- *In* comes from the Latin word "in," meaning not.
- *Continence* comes from the Latin word "continentia," meaning holding together.

10. **Macular**

- Comes from the Latin word "macula," meaning spot or stain.

11. **Degeneration**

- Comes from the Latin word "degenerare," meaning to decline from an ancestral standard.

12. **Hearing**

- Comes from the Old English word "hieran," not directly from Latin or Greek.

13. **Osteoarthritis**

- *Osteo* comes from the Greek word "osteon" (ὀστέον), meaning bone.
- *Arthritis* as mentioned above.

14. **Therapy**

- Comes from the Greek word "therapeia" (θεραπεία), meaning healing or medical treatment.

15. **Cognitive**

- Comes from the Latin word "cognitio," meaning knowing or learning.

TASK 5: MAKE A CHOICE

1. What is a primary focus of geriatric medicine?

A) Pediatric care

B) Sports injuries

C) Health conditions affecting older adults

D) Infectious diseases in young adults

2. Cardiovascular diseases in the elderly often manifest as:

A) Joint pain and stiffness

B) Shortness of breath, chest pain, and dizziness

C) Memory loss and confusion

D) Increased thirst and frequent urination

3. Effective management of hypertension typically involves:

A) Cognitive therapy

B) Lifestyle modifications and medication

C) Surgery

D) High-intensity exercise

4. Arthritis in older adults is characterized by:

A) High fever and rash

B) Joint pain, stiffness, and swelling

C) Frequent urination and thirst

D) Severe respiratory problems

5. Which is NOT a management strategy for arthritis?

A) Physical therapy B) Pain relief medications

C) High-impact exercises D) Surgical interventions

6. Osteoporosis is often detected:

A) During routine physical exams

B) After a fracture occurs

C) Through specific blood tests

D) Via genetic screening

7. The management of osteoporosis includes:

A) High carbohydrate diet

B) Calcium and vitamin D supplements

C) Frequent high-impact activities

D) Avoidance of sunlight

8. Alzheimer's Disease and dementia are characterized by:

A) Joint pain and inflammation

B) Memory loss and difficulty with communication

C) Frequent urination and thirst

D) Shortness of breath and chest pain

9. Diabetes in older adults is indicated by symptoms like:

A) Increased thirst, frequent urination, and blurred vision

B) Memory loss and disorientation

C) Persistent cough and wheezing

D) Severe joint pain and swelling

10. COPD management includes:

A) Smoking cessation and pulmonary rehabilitation

B) Intense cardiovascular exercises

C) Calcium and vitamin D supplements

D) High carbohydrate diet

11. What is a common symptom of geriatric depression?

A) Joint inflammation

B) Persistent sadness and loss of interest in activities

C) Blurred vision

D) Frequent bone fractures

12. Urinary incontinence in older adults is managed with:

A) High-impact exercises

B) Pelvic floor exercises and bladder training

C) Cognitive therapy

D) High carbohydrate diet

13. Age-Related Macular Degeneration primarily affects:

A) Memory and cognitive function

B) The joints and bones

C) Central vision

D) The respiratory system

14. A common symptom of hearing loss in the elderly is:

A) Difficulty hearing conversations, especially in noisy environments

B) Frequent urination

C) Severe joint pain

D) Persistent sadness and loss of interest

15. Key to managing many geriatric diseases is:

A) High-intensity exercise and a high carbohydrate diet

B) Early detection and regular monitoring

C) Surgery and high-impact activities

D) Isolation and reduced social interaction

Chapter 18: Hospice and Terminal Care

Hospice and end-of-life care are essential components of healthcare that focus on providing comfort and dignity to patients facing terminal illnesses. This specialized care prioritizes the quality of life for patients in their final days, ensuring their physical, emotional, and spiritual needs are met compassionately. This article delves into the principles of hospice care and its importance for terminal patients and their families.

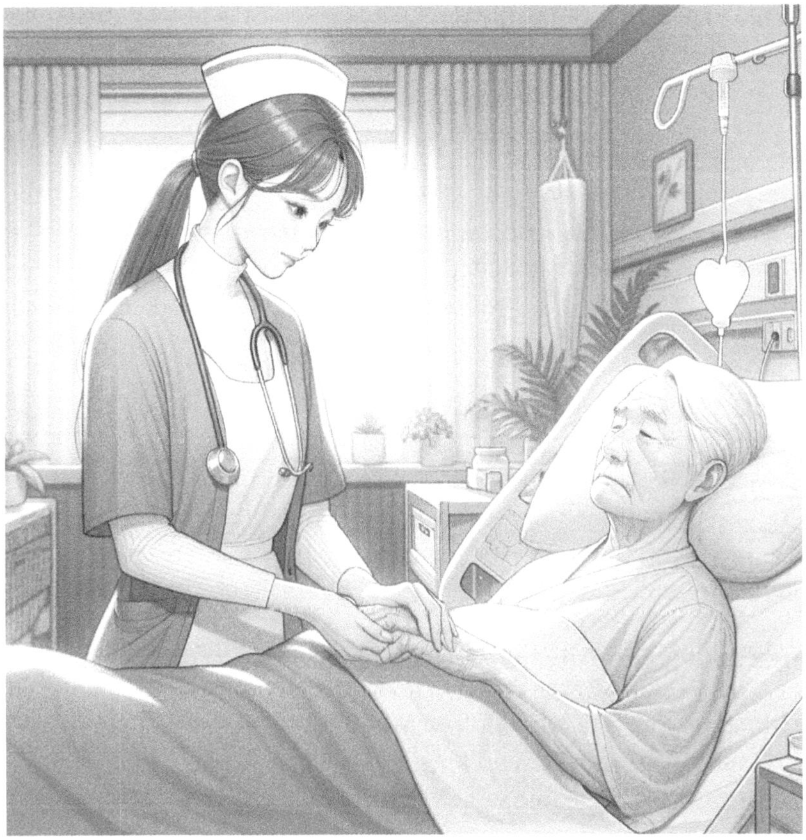

Understanding Hospice Care

Hospice care is a holistic approach that aims to alleviate suffering and improve the quality of life for patients who have a limited life expectancy, typically six months or less. Unlike curative treatments, hospice focuses on palliative care—relieving symptoms without curing the underlying disease. The goal is to provide a peaceful, comfortable, and dignified end-of-life experience.

The Hospice Team

A unique aspect of hospice care is the interdisciplinary team approach. This team usually includes doctors, nurses, social workers, spiritual advisors, and trained volunteers. They work collaboratively to address the physical, emotional, spiritual, and practical needs of the patient and their family.

1. **Medical Care**: Pain management and symptom control are at the forefront of hospice medical care. The medical team closely monitors the patient to provide relief from pain, breathlessness, and other distressing symptoms.
2. **Emotional and Psychological Support**: Social workers and counselors offer emotional support to patients and families, helping them cope with the challenges of terminal illness.
3. **Spiritual Care**: Spiritual advisors or chaplains provide comfort and guidance according to the patient's beliefs and preferences, helping them find peace and meaning in their final days.
4. **Family Support**: Hospice also extends support to the family, offering counseling, bereavement support, and help with practical matters like planning and caregiving.

The Role of Palliative Care

Palliative care, integral to hospice, focuses on providing relief from the symptoms and stress of a serious illness. It can be provided alongside curative treatments before transitioning fully to hospice care. Palliative care specialists work in conjunction with other healthcare providers to offer an extra layer of support.

Home-Based Hospice vs. Facility Care

Hospice care can be provided in various settings. Many patients prefer home-based hospice, as it allows them to remain in a familiar and comfortable environment. However, hospice facilities, hospitals, and nursing homes can also provide hospice care, particularly when complex medical attention is required.

Decision Making and Advance Directives

End-of-life care involves crucial decision-making about the patient's care preferences. Advance directives, such as living wills and healthcare proxies, help ensure that a patient's wishes are respected even if they become unable to communicate their decisions.

The Importance of Bereavement Support

Hospice care extends beyond the patient's death, offering bereavement support to families. Grief counseling, support groups, and resources are provided to help loved ones navigate their loss and begin the healing process.

Hospice and end-of-life care play a vital role in the healthcare system, providing compassionate care that honors the dignity and wishes of terminal patients. By focusing on comfort rather than cure, hospice helps patients and their families experience a more peaceful and meaningful end-of-life journey. It stands as a testament to the belief that every stage of human life, including its end, should be treated with care, respect, and dignity.

TASK 1: FILL IN THE BLANKS

1. Hospice care aims to alleviate suffering and improve the __________ for patients with limited life expectancy.
2. Unlike curative treatments, hospice focuses on __________ care.
3. The hospice team typically includes doctors, nurses, __________ workers, spiritual advisors, and volunteers.
4. A key aspect of medical care in hospice is __________ management and symptom control.
5. Emotional and psychological support in hospice care helps patients and families cope with the __________ of terminal illness.
6. Spiritual advisors in hospice provide comfort according to the patient's __________ and preferences.
7. Hospice care also offers bereavement support and help with __________ matters for families.
8. __________ care, integral to hospice, provides relief from symptoms and stress of a serious illness.
9. Many patients prefer __________-based hospice, allowing them to stay in a familiar environment.
10. Advance __________, like living wills, ensure a patient's care preferences are respected.
11. After a patient's death, hospice provides __________ support to families.
12. Hospice care stands as a testament to the belief that every stage of human life should be treated with __________, respect, and dignity.

TASK 2: LET'S TALK

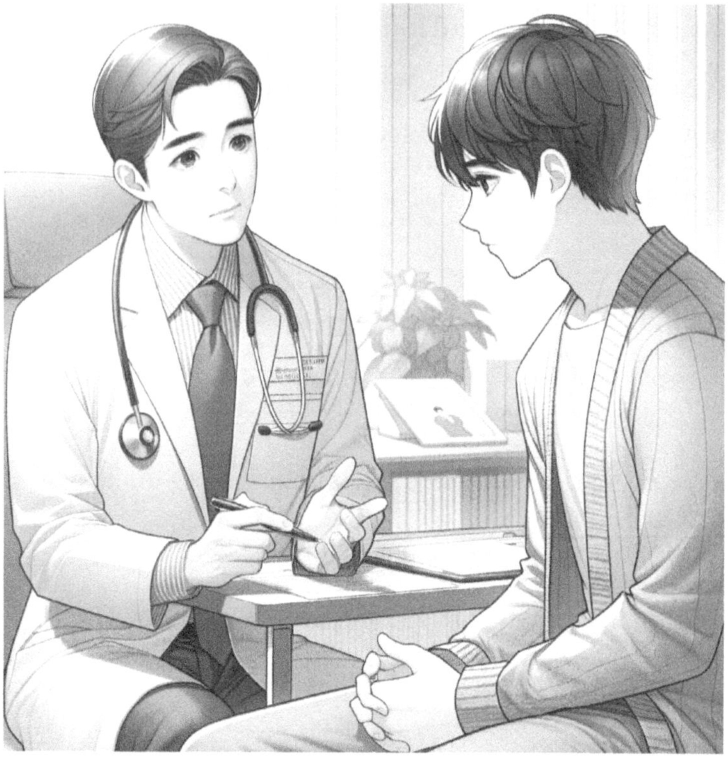

Nurse: Good afternoon, I'm Nurse Thompson. I understand that this is a challenging time for you and your family. We're here to ensure your father receives the best care in his final days.

Son: Thank you, Nurse Thompson. We just want to make sure his last days are as comfortable as possible. He's expressed some final wishes…

Nurse: Absolutely, we respect and prioritize fulfilling his last wishes. Could you share what he has expressed?

Son: Well, he's always loved classical music. He wishes to listen to his favorite compositions during his final days. And he's a devout man, he'd like to have someone to read bible verses

Nurse: We can certainly arrange for that. We believe in catering to the emotional and spiritual needs of our patients as much as their physical comfort. Our hospice has access to a library of music, and we can play his favorite compositions in his room. As for spiritual support, I'll coordinate with our staff to schedule regular visits with a staff member to read to him.

Son: That would mean a lot to him, and to us. How do you manage his physical comfort?

Nurse: Our primary goal is to manage any pain or discomfort he might be experiencing. Our medical team will closely monitor his condition to administer appropriate pain management and symptom control medications. We'll ensure he's as comfortable and pain-free as possible.

Son: What about his nutrition and other needs?

Nurse: We'll provide nutrition as tolerated and preferred by him. Our staff will assist with all his basic needs, ensuring he is well-cared for. We also encourage family members to spend as much time with their loved ones as they wish.

Son: We're worried about after... when he's gone. How do we handle that?

Nurse: We understand how difficult this time is for families. Our hospice provides bereavement support services, including counseling and support groups. We're here to support you and your family through the grieving process as well.

Son: Thank you. Knowing there's a support system for both him and us is very reassuring.

Nurse: It's our privilege to provide this care. Remember, we are here to support you every step of the way. If you have any more questions or specific requests, please don't hesitate to ask.

TASK 3: DO YOU REMEMBER

1. **What is the primary aim of hospice care for patients with limited life expectancy?**

____

____

____

2. **What type of care does hospice focus on, which is different from curative treatments?**

____

____

____

3. **Name two professionals typically included in the interdisciplinary hospice care team.**

____

____

____

4. **What is a key aspect of medical care in hospice?**

____

____

____

5. **Why is emotional and psychological support important in hospice care?**

6. **How does hospice care address the spiritual needs of patients?**

7. **What type of support does hospice care extend to the families of patients?**

8. **What is the role of palliative care in the context of hospice?**

9. **What are advance directives, and why are they important in hospice care?**

10. **What support does hospice provide to families after the patient's death?**

TASK 4: LATIN AND GREEK TIME

1. **Hospice**

    - Derived from the Latin word "hospitium," meaning hospitality or the care of strangers.

2. **Terminal**

    - Comes from the Latin word "terminalis," meaning pertaining to a boundary or end.

3. **Palliative**

    - Originates from the Latin word "palliare," meaning to cloak or cover, referring to relieving symptoms without curing the underlying disease.

4. **Interdisciplinary**

    - *Inter* comes from the Latin word "inter," meaning between or among.
    - *Disciplinary* comes from the Latin word "disciplina," meaning instruction or knowledge.

5. **Psychological**

    - *Psycho* comes from the Greek word "psyche" (ψυχή), meaning soul or mind.
    - *Logical* comes from the Greek word "logikos" (λογικός), meaning pertaining to reason or speech.

6. **Nutrition**

    - Comes from the Latin word "nutritio," meaning nourishing or the act of feeding.

7. **Bereavement**

    - Derived from the Old English word "bereafian," meaning to deprive or take away, not directly from Latin or Greek.

8. **Counseling**

    - Originates from the Old French word "conseil," meaning advice, not directly from Latin or Greek.

9. **Symptom**

    - Comes from the Greek word "symptoma" (σύμπτωμα), meaning an occurrence or happenstance.

10. **Pain Management**

    - *Pain* comes from the Latin word "poena," meaning penalty or punishment.

- *Management* comes from the Latin word "manu agere," meaning to lead by the hand.

11. **Emotional**

- Derived from the Latin word "emovere," meaning to move out or stir up.

12. **Spiritual**

- Comes from the Latin word "spiritualis," meaning of or pertaining to breath, spirit.

13. **Dignity**

- Originates from the Latin word "dignitas," meaning worthiness or honor.

14. **Therapy**

- Comes from the Greek word "therapeia" (θεραπεία), meaning healing or medical treatment.

TASK 5: MAKE A CHOICE

1. What is the primary focus of hospice care?

A) Curative treatment B) Palliative care

C) Surgical interventions D) Diagnostic testing

2. Hospice care primarily aims to improve what aspect for terminal patients?

A) Financial stability B) Longevity of life

C) Quality of life D) Physical fitness

3. Which of the following professionals is typically not part of a hospice care team?

A) Social worker B) Spiritual advisor

C) Financial advisor D) Nurse

4. What is a key aspect of medical care in hospice?

A) Aggressive treatment

B) Pain management and symptom control

C) Frequent surgeries

D) Intensive physiotherapy

5. Palliative care in the context of hospice primarily focuses on:

A) Providing a cure for the illness

B) Relieving symptoms and reducing stress

C) Conducting extensive medical research

D) Implementing rigorous physical therapy

6. What is the role of a spiritual advisor in hospice care?

A) Provide financial advice

B) Administer medications

C) Offer comfort and guidance based on patient's beliefs

D) Conduct physical examinations

7. Advance directives in hospice care are important for:

A) Financial planning

B) Ensuring patient's care preferences are respected

C) Arranging post-mortem services

D) Legal documentation purposes only

8. Which setting is not a common place for providing hospice care?

A) Patient's home B) Hospice facility

C) Hospital D) Corporate offices

9. After a patient's death, hospice care provides:

A) Legal support B) Bereavement support

C) Financial loans D) Employment counseling

10. Which is not a typical characteristic of hospice care?

A) Interdisciplinary team approach

B) Focus on the family's physical health

C) Emotional and psychological support

D) Management of pain and symptoms

Chapter 19: Medical Ethics

Medical ethics forms the backbone of healthcare practices, ensuring that medical professionals, particularly nurses, adhere to principles that safeguard patient well-being and dignity. This article delves into the depth of medical ethics in nursing, exploring the historical context and contemporary relevance of ethical oaths, and examining the catastrophic consequences of ethical breaches, as evidenced during the Nazi regime.

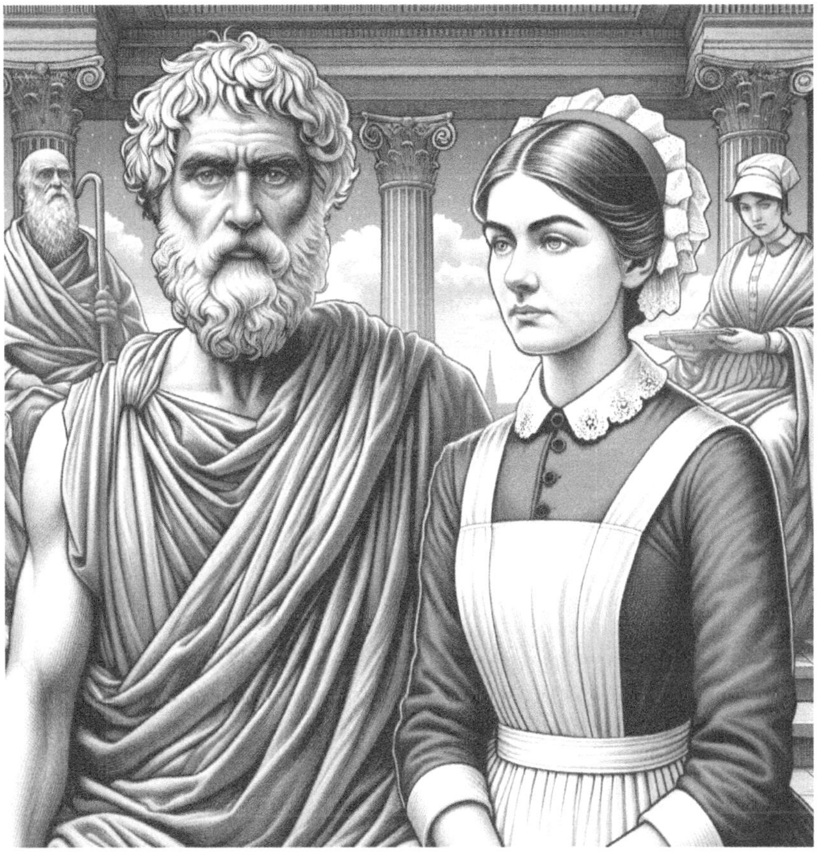

MEDICAL ETHICS: A PILLAR OF HEALTHCARE

Medical ethics refers to the set of moral principles that govern the behavior of healthcare professionals. It encompasses more than just the Hippocratic and Nightingale Oaths; it includes a range of legal regulations specific to each country. Nurses are expected to not only obey these laws but also employ their moral judgment in complex situations.

THE HIPPOCRATIC OATH

Originating in ancient Greece, the Hippocratic Oath is one of the oldest binding documents in history. Traditionally taken by physicians, it lays down ethical standards for practicing medicine. Key tenets include the obligation to respect patient privacy, treat the sick to the best of one's ability, preserve patient autonomy, and most importantly, "do no harm" (non-maleficence).

THE NIGHTINGALE OATH

Named after Florence Nightingale, the founder of modern nursing, this oath is a statement of the ethics and principles of the nursing profession. It emphasizes the commitment to personal integrity, confidentiality in patient care, and dedication to patient health. It serves as a reminder to nurses of their commitment to compassionate care, lifelong learning, and professional accountability.

LEGAL REGULATIONS

Each country has its own set of laws governing medical practices, which nurses must adhere to. These laws are designed to protect patient rights and ensure the delivery of safe, ethical, and competent care.

ETHICS IN CLINICAL PRACTICE

Nurses face a myriad of ethical considerations in clinical practice:

- **Patient Autonomy**: This principle emphasizes the right of patients to make decisions about their medical care without undue influence from healthcare providers. It includes respecting patients' cultural and religious beliefs, as seen in scenarios where patients refuse certain treatments like blood transfusions.

- **Confidentiality**: Essential to the nurse-patient relationship, confidentiality involves keeping personal health information private unless consent to disclose is given.

- **Informed Consent**: This is a critical process that involves informing patients about the risks and benefits of treatments and ensuring they understand and consent to them.

- **End-of-Life Decisions**: Nurses often guide patients through complex decisions about end-of-life care. This includes respecting patients' wishes and ensuring their choices are honored.

THE DARK CHAPTER OF MEDICAL ETHICS: NAZI ERA BREACHES

The Nazi period stands as a grim reminder of the catastrophic consequences of ethical violations:

- **Aktion T4 Program**: A policy of involuntary euthanasia, this program led to the systematic killing of individuals deemed "unworthy of life," including those with disabilities or chronic illnesses.

- **Human Experimentation**: Under the guise of medical research, horrific experiments were conducted on concentration camp prisoners without consent. These included exposure to infectious diseases, sterilization, and testing the limits of human endurance.

- **Notorious Figures**: Individuals like Josef Mengele conducted inhumane experiments, particularly on twins, in an attempt to advance racial and genetic ideology.

The Nuremberg Trials post-World War II formulated the Nuremberg Code, setting the foundation for modern research ethics, emphasizing voluntary consent, and the right to withdraw from experiments.

CONTEMPORARY RELEVANCE OF MEDICAL ETHICS

In the modern healthcare landscape, medical ethics continues to play a critical role:

- **Professional Conduct**: Nurses must navigate ethical dilemmas daily, balancing patient care needs with ethical principles.
- **Legal Implications**: Understanding and adhering to the legal aspects of medical ethics is vital. Breaches can lead to malpractice allegations and erosion of public trust.
- **Cultural Competence**: In an increasingly diverse society, nurses must be culturally sensitive, respecting different health beliefs and practices.

Medical ethics is not just a theoretical concept but a practical guide that shapes every aspect of nursing care. From the commitment encapsulated in the Hippocratic and Nightingale Oaths to the legal and moral obligations nurses uphold, medical ethics is integral to the profession. The harrowing lessons from the Nazi era underscore the importance of unwavering adherence to these ethical standards. In essence, medical ethics is central to maintaining the integrity, trust, and professionalism of nursing, ensuring that patient care remains compassionate, safe, and effective.

TASK 1: FILL IN THE BLANKS

1. Medical ethics is a set of __________ principles governing the behavior of healthcare professionals.
2. The __________ Oath, originating in ancient Greece, emphasizes the principle of "do no harm."
3. The __________ Oath is named after the founder of modern nursing and emphasizes commitment to patient care.
4. Nurses must adhere to legal __________ specific to each country while practicing.
5. __________ autonomy is the right of patients to make decisions about their medical care without undue influence.
6. Maintaining patient __________ is a crucial aspect of the nurse-patient relationship.
7. Informed __________ involves educating patients about the risks and benefits of treatments and ensuring their understanding.
8. The __________ T4 Program during the Nazi era involved involuntary euthanasia of individuals deemed unfit.

9. The horrific __________ experiments during the Nazi regime violated fundamental ethical principles.

10. The __________ Code, formulated post-World War II, set the foundation for modern research ethics.

11. Ethical dilemmas in nursing often involve balancing patient care needs with __________ principles.

12. Understanding legal aspects of medical ethics is vital to avoid __________ allegations.

13. Nurses must demonstrate __________ competence, respecting diverse health beliefs and practices.

14. The two oaths that guide medical ethics in nursing are the Hippocratic and __________ Oaths.

15. The article highlights the importance of medical ethics in maintaining the __________, trust, and professionalism of nursing.

TASK 2: LET'S TALK

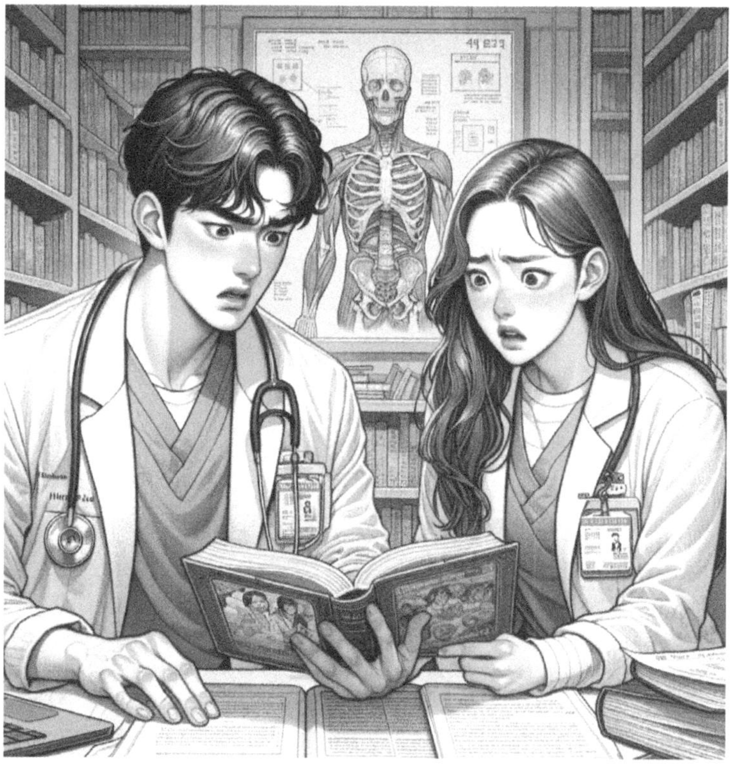

Maya: Hey Ben, after reading about medical ethics in nursing, I've been thinking a lot about how crucial our moral responsibility is.

Ben: Absolutely, Maya. It's not just about skills and knowledge, but also about upholding ethical principles. The Hippocratic Oath and the Nightingale Oath really emphasize our commitment to doing no harm and respecting patient autonomy.

Maya: Exactly. And when I read about the Nazi doctors and nurses and how they betrayed their patients, it was horrifying. It's unthinkable how they completely abandoned their ethical duties.

Ben: I know, it's chilling. The Aktion T4 program and the human experiments... it's a stark reminder of why our ethical codes are so important. It shows the worst of what can happen when medical professionals lose their moral compass.

Maya: It makes me even more determined to be ethical in my practice. Patient confidentiality, informed consent, and respecting their rights are principles I want to always stand by.

Ben: Same here. And it's not just about following laws and regulations; it's about using our conscience to make decisions, especially in complex situations.

Maya: Exactly! Like dealing with end-of-life decisions or respecting patients' cultural and religious beliefs. These situations require us to be not only knowledgeable but also empathetic and morally grounded.

Ben: Right. And I think being aware of different cultural perspectives is crucial. We're going to encounter patients from diverse backgrounds, and being culturally competent is a part of being ethical.

Maya: True. I think being ethical also means being professional and avoiding any form of negligence or misconduct. We have a duty to our patients to provide the best care possible.

Ben: Absolutely. I believe that as future nurses, we have the power to make a positive impact on our patients' lives. Staying true to our ethical principles is how we honor that responsibility.

Maya: Agreed, Ben. It's a big responsibility, but I'm ready for it. We're going to be great nurses who make a real difference.

TASK 3: DO YOU REMEMBER?

1. **What does medical ethics in healthcare primarily ensure?**

____

____

____

2. **Besides the Hippocratic and Nightingale Oaths, what else does medical ethics in nursing include?**

____

____

____

3. **From which ancient civilization does the Hippocratic Oath originate?**

4. **What is one of the key tenets of the Hippocratic Oath regarding patient treatment?**

5. **Who is the Nightingale Oath named after?**

6. **What does the Nightingale Oath emphasize in the nursing profession?**

7. **What is the purpose of legal regulations in medical practices that nurses must adhere to?**

8. **What principle in medical ethics emphasizes the right of patients to make their own medical decisions?**

9. **Why is confidentiality essential in the nurse-patient relationship?**

10. **What critical process involves informing patients about the risks and benefits of treatments?**

11. **What role do nurses often play in guiding patients through end-of-life decisions?**

12. **During the Nazi era, what was the Aktion T4 Program?**

13. **What type of unethical practices were conducted under human experimentation during the Nazi regime?**

14. **What was established post-World War II to set the foundation for modern research ethics?**

15. **In contemporary healthcare, why is cultural competence important for nurses?**

____

TASK 4: LATIN AND GREEK TIME

1. **Medical**
   - Comes from the Latin word "medicus," meaning physician or medicine.
2. **Ethics**
   - Derived from the Greek word "ethos" (ἦθος), meaning character or custom.
3. **Hippocratic**
   - Named after Hippocrates, from the Greek name "Hippokrates" (Ἱπποκράτης), meaning horse power.
4. **Oath**
   - Comes from the Old English word "āþ," not directly from Latin or Greek.
5. **Nightingale**
   - Named after Florence Nightingale; the term 'nightingale' itself comes from Old English but is not directly of Latin or Greek origin.
6. **Autonomy**
   - *Auto* comes from the Greek word "autos" (αὐτός), meaning self.
   - *Nomy* comes from the Greek word "nomos" (νόμος), meaning law or custom.
7. **Confidentiality**
   - Derived from the Latin word "confidentialis," meaning something entrusted with faith.
8. **Consent**
   - Comes from the Latin word "consentire," meaning feel together.
9. **Euthanasia**

- *Eu* comes from the Greek word "eu" (εὖ), meaning good.
- *Thanasia* comes from the Greek word "thanatos" (θάνατος), meaning death.

10. **Experimentation**
    - Derived from the Latin word "experimentum," meaning trial or test.
11. **Nuremberg**
    - Refers to the city of Nuremberg in Germany, not derived from Latin or Greek.
12. **Code**
    - Comes from the Latin word "codex," meaning book or system of laws.
13. **Professional**
    - Derived from the Latin word "professio," meaning public declaration.
14. **Legal**
    - Comes from the Latin word "legalis," meaning pertaining to the law.
15. **Cultural**
    - Derived from the Latin word "cultura," meaning cultivation or education.

TASK 5: MAKE A CHOICE

1. Medical ethics in healthcare primarily ensures:

   A) Financial profitability

   B) Technological advancement

   C) Patient well-being and dignity

   D) Hospital administration efficiency

2. Besides the Hippocratic and Nightingale Oaths, medical ethics in nursing also includes:

   A) Astrological beliefs

   B) A range of legal regulations

C) Personal opinions of nurses

D) Traditional healing practices

3. The Hippocratic Oath originated from:

A) Ancient Rome B) Ancient Greece

C) Medieval Europe D) Ancient Egypt

4. A key tenet of the Hippocratic Oath is:

A) To guarantee a cure B) To perform surgery

C) "Do no harm" D) To prescribe medication

5. The Nightingale Oath is named after:

A) Florence Henderson B) Florence Griffith Joyner

C) Florence Nightingale D) Florence Welch

6. The Nightingale Oath emphasizes in nursing:

A) Personal integrity and patient health

B) Financial management skills

C) Research and development

D) Political awareness

7. Legal regulations in medical practices are designed to:

A) Increase hospital revenue

B) Protect patient rights

C) Promote pharmaceutical products

D) Limit the power of nurses

8. Patient autonomy in medical ethics emphasizes:

A) The nurse's decision-making authority

B) The patient's right to make their own medical decisions

C) The family's wishes over the patient's

D) Government policies on healthcare

9. The Aktion T4 Program during the Nazi era was a policy of:

A) Free healthcare for all

B) Involuntary euthanasia

C) Community health education

D) Medical research grants

10. The Nuremberg Code, established post-World War II, set the foundation for:

A) Modern surgical techniques

B) Hospital administrative procedures

C) Modern research ethics

D) Nursing education curricula

Chapter 20 :Teamwork

In the dynamic setting of a hospital, effective teamwork among nurses and other healthcare professionals is pivotal for delivering high-quality patient care. The ability to collaborate and communicate efficiently within and across teams is an essential aspect of nursing, serving as a bridge between doctors, patients, and the hospital.

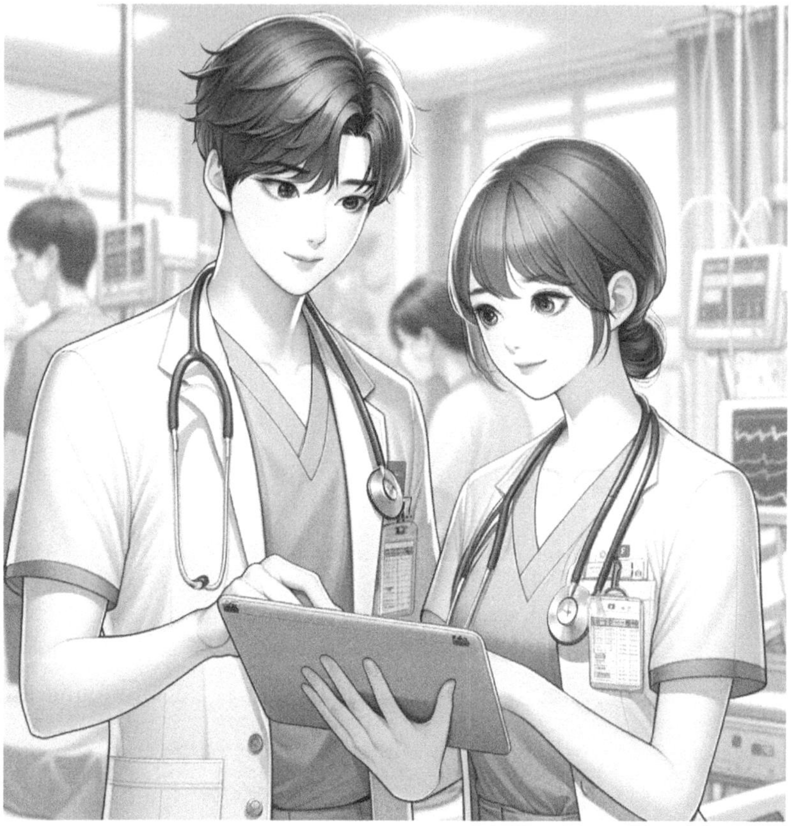

The Importance of Teamwork and Collaboration

The World Health Organization (WHO) highlights that effective teamwork in healthcare can significantly enhance patient safety. Modern healthcare rarely involves just one medical professional; therefore, teamwork and coordination are vital to minimize adverse events stemming from communication errors and misunderstandings of professional roles.

Distinction Between Teamwork and Collaboration

While often used interchangeably, teamwork and collaboration have subtle differences in the context of nursing. Collaboration refers to joint efforts between various teams or groups. For instance, a cardiac surgery team might collaborate with the maternity ward to care for a pregnant patient with heart issues. Teamwork, on the other hand, focuses on the efforts within a single team to yield the best outcomes.

Strategies for Enhancing Teamwork and Collaboration

1. **Establish Team Goals**: Setting clear, common goals like improving patient care or shortening response times helps unify the team and provides a direction for collective efforts.
2. **Assign Roles Within a Team**: Understanding key roles within teams ensures better collaboration. Clear role assignments prevent duplication of efforts and ensure no aspect of patient care is overlooked.
3. **Allow for Open Communication**: Effective communication is critical. Encouraging active listening and acknowledging team members' input fosters a cohesive and efficient work environment.
4. **Promote Mutual Respect**: Respect is crucial in healthcare settings. A team where each member feels valued is more likely to be engaged and collaborative.
5. **Handle Conflict Proactively**: Recognizing that conflict is inevitable and addressing it early through open communication can prevent escalation and maintain team harmony.
6. **Be an Effective Leader**: Leadership in nursing isn't just about managing tasks; it's about fostering a supportive and adaptable team environment.

Benefits of Teamwork in Nursing

Effective teamwork in nursing leads to numerous benefits, including:

- **Greater Job Satisfaction**: Good teamwork reduces stress and increases workplace happiness, leading to a balanced workload.
- **Improved Patient Care**: Collaborative care results in consistent standards and safer treatment processes.
- **More Efficient Processes**: Effective delegation and teamwork save time and enhance the quality of patient care.
- **Stronger Professional Connections**: Teamwork strengthens professional networks and opens up opportunities for mentorship and career development.
- **Lower Healthcare Costs**: Efficient teamwork can lead to more cost-effective use of resources.
- **Improved Regulatory Compliance**: Enhanced oversight and accountability contribute to better adherence to healthcare regulations.

Tips for Improving Teamwork as a Nurse

1. **Increase Communication**: Foster open communication for better collaboration and improved patient outcomes.
2. **Be Transparent**: Transparency ensures everyone on the team is on the same page, fostering trust and clarity.

3. **Clarify Roles**: Clear role definitions enable smoother team operations and efficient task completion.

4. **Promote Adaptability**: Being adaptable allows nurses to respond effectively to changing situations and patient needs.

5. **Follow Up**: Regular follow-ups with healthcare providers and colleagues ensure tasks are completed and goals are met.

6. **Complete Regular Training**: Ongoing professional development keeps the team up-to-date and strengthens collective skills.

7. **Set an Example**: Leading by example cultivates a culture of teamwork and collaboration.

In the hospital and nursing environments, teamwork and collaboration are not just ideals but necessities for ensuring patient safety and care. By establishing clear goals, fostering open communication, and promoting mutual respect, nursing teams can function more cohesively and effectively. The benefits of such an approach extend beyond patient care, enhancing job satisfaction, professional growth, and overall healthcare delivery.

TASK 1: FILL IN THE BLANKS

1. The World Health Organization emphasizes that effective teamwork in healthcare can significantly improve __________.

2. In nursing, collaboration refers to joint efforts between __________, while teamwork focuses on efforts within __________.

3. One key strategy for enhancing teamwork is to __________ within a team.

4. Assigning __________ helps prevent duplication of efforts and ensures comprehensive patient care.

5. Open __________ is crucial for effective teamwork, involving active listening and acknowledging team members' input.

6. Mutual __________ among team members is critical for a cohesive working environment.

7. Proactive __________ management is essential in maintaining team harmony and effectiveness.

8. An effective leader in nursing should foster a __________ and __________ team environment.

9. Good teamwork in nursing leads to greater __________ and __________.

10. Improved __________ is a benefit of effective teamwork and collaboration in nursing.

11. Teamwork helps in lowering overall __________ in healthcare.

12. To improve teamwork skills, nurses should focus on increasing __________ among team members.

13. Being __________ with nursing colleagues and patients promotes better teamwork.

14. Regular __________ training can enhance the nursing team's skills and knowledge.

15. Setting a good __________ in the team can encourage a culture of collaboration and teamwork.

TASK 2: LET'S TALK

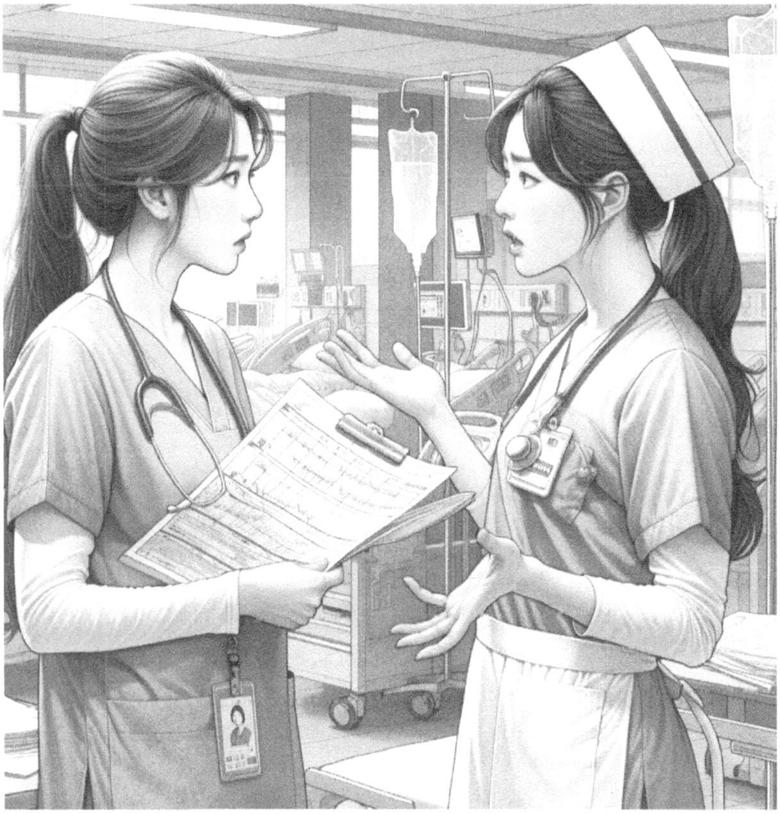

Nurse 1 (Emma): [Anxiously] Sarah, why didn't you update the patient's chart? Dr. Smith was asking for it, and now there's confusion about the medication dosage!

Nurse 2 (Sarah): [Defensively] I was swamped with emergencies in the other ward. I thought you were going to do it since you were on duty here!

Emma: But communication is key, Sarah! We can't just assume things in such critical situations.

Sarah: I know, I know. It's just... everything was happening at once. I should have informed you. I'm sorry.

Emma: [Taking a deep breath] I understand, it's been incredibly hectic. I'm sorry for snapping at you. It's just the pressure…

Sarah: I get it. We're both under a lot of stress. Let's figure out a system to avoid this in the future. What about a quick handover meeting during shift changes?

Emma: That's a good idea. Also, we could use a shared digital log for updates. It might be more efficient and transparent.

Sarah: Agreed. And we should definitely clarify our roles for each shift. I think part of the issue was the overlap and confusion about who was handling what.

Emma: Right, like they mentioned in our last team meeting about the importance of role clarity. We should put that into practice.

Sarah: Absolutely. And let's make sure we both have a chance to voice any concerns during our shift. Open communication is key, as you said.

Emma: Definitely. And mutual respect. We're both here for the same reason - to provide the best care for our patients. We're a team, after all.

Sarah: Exactly. Thanks for understanding, Emma. I really appreciate it.

Emma: Same here, Sarah. Let's continue to support each other. Our teamwork can make all the difference in this high-pressure environment.

Sarah: Agreed. Let's report this incident and our resolution to our supervisor. It might be helpful for the whole team to learn from this.

Emma: Great idea. We're stronger when we work together and learn from our mistakes.

TASK 3: DO YOU REMEMBER?

1. **According to the WHO, what significant impact can effective teamwork in healthcare have?**

____

____

____

2. **What does collaboration in a nursing context specifically refer to?**

____

____

____

3. **In the context of the article, what is the difference between teamwork and collaboration in nursing?**

4. **What is a key strategy mentioned in the article for enhancing teamwork?**

5. **Why is assigning clear roles within a team important in a nursing environment?**

6. **What type of communication is crucial for effective teamwork in nursing, as per the article?**

7. **How is mutual respect important in creating a cohesive working environment in healthcare?**

8. **In the conversation, what problem did Nurse Emma and Nurse Sarah encounter?**

9. **What solution did Nurse Emma and Nurse Sarah agree upon to prevent future misunderstandings?**

10. **Why did Nurse Emma apologize to Nurse Sarah in their conversation?**

11. **What did Nurse Sarah suggest for better shift changeovers?**

12. **According to the article, what role does leadership play in nursing teamwork?**

13. **What are two benefits of effective teamwork in nursing mentioned in the article?**

14. **How can regular training enhance a nursing team's effectiveness?**

15. **In the conversation, what did the nurses decide to do to contribute to team learning and improvement?**

TASK 4: LATIN AND GREEK TIME

1. **Hospital**

   - Comes from the Latin word "hospes," meaning guest or host.

2. **Teamwork**

   - *Team* comes from the Old English word "tēam," meaning a group of draft animals, not directly from Latin or Greek.
   - *Work* comes from the Old English word "weorc," not directly from Latin or Greek.

3. **Collaboration**

   - Derived from the Latin word "collaborare," meaning to work together.

4. **Communication**

   - Comes from the Latin word "communicare," meaning to share or make common.

5. **Organization**

   - Derived from the Greek word "organon" (ὄργανον), meaning instrument or tool.

6. **Healthcare**

   - *Health* comes from the Old English word "hælþ," not directly from Latin or Greek.
   - *Care* comes from the Old English word "caru," meaning sorrow or anxiety, not directly from Latin or Greek.

7. **Professional**

   - Derived from the Latin word "professio," meaning declaration or public claim.

8. **Leadership**

   - Comes from the Old English word "lædan," meaning to lead, not directly from Latin or Greek.

9. **Regulatory**

   - Derived from the Latin word "regulare," meaning to control by rule.

10. **Transparency**

- Comes from the Latin word "transparens," meaning shining through.

11. **Adaptability**

- Derived from the Latin word "adaptare," meaning to fit or adjust.

12. **Training**

- Comes from the Old French word "trainer," meaning to drag or draw, not directly from Latin or Greek.

13. **Efficiency**

- Derived from the Latin word "efficientia," meaning effectiveness.

14. **Compliance**

- Comes from the Latin word "complere," meaning to fill up or complete.

TASK 5: MAKE A CHOICE

1. What is essential for delivering high-quality patient care in a hospital setting?

A) Competition among nurses

B) Effective teamwork among healthcare professionals

C) Individual performance

D) Technology-driven solutions

2. Effective teamwork in healthcare is crucial for:

A) Reducing financial costs only

B) Enhancing patient safety

C) Increasing hospital reputation

D) Simplifying administrative tasks

3. According to the article, what does collaboration in nursing refer to?

A) Working independently

B) Joint efforts between various teams or groups

C) Following instructions without questioning

D) Avoiding team interactions

4. What is a key strategy for enhancing teamwork and collaboration?

A) Establishing team goals

B) Reducing team size

C) Limiting communication

D) Focusing on individual achievements

5. In the context of nursing, promoting mutual respect is important for:

A) Creating a competitive environment

B) Ensuring a team where each member feels valued

C) Reducing the need for communication

D) Increasing individual autonomy

6. What can effective delegation and teamwork lead to in nursing?

A) More efficient processes

B) Decreased job satisfaction

C) Reduced patient interaction

D) Increased healthcare costs

7. How can nurses improve teamwork?

A) By reducing transparency

B) By promoting open communication

C) By avoiding regular training

D) By focusing solely on clinical skills

8. What is a benefit of effective teamwork in nursing?

A) Reduced job satisfaction

B) Stronger professional connections

C) Limited patient care options

D) Increased workload for individual nurses

9. Regular follow-ups with healthcare providers and colleagues ensure:

A) Tasks are completed and goals are met

B) Less need for team meetings

C) Decreased accountability

D) Increased administrative work

10. The article suggests that teamwork and collaboration in nursing are:

A) Optional preferences

B) Necessities for ensuring patient safety and care

C) Only important in large hospitals

D) Less effective than individual work

Bibliography

Naude, Alaric (2019) "Introduction to Mammalian and Human Dimorphism: A Biological Approach to Understanding True Masculinity and Femininity" - New Male Studies - An International Journal (AIMHS- Australian Institute of Male Health & Studies)

Johnson, W; Bouchard Jr., Thomas J. (2005-07-01). "The structure of human intelligence: It is verbal, perceptual, and image rotation (VPR), not fluid and crystallized". Intelligence. 33 (4): 393– 416. doi:10.1016/j.intell.2004.12.002.

Jensen, A.R. (1980). "Bias in mental testing." New York: Free Press. Jensen, A. R., & Reynolds, C. R. (1983), Sex differences on the WISC-R. Personality and Individual Differences, 4, 223-226.

Lynn, R., & Irwing, P. (2004). "Sex differences on the progressive matrices: A meta-analysis." Intelligence, 32(5), 481-498

Rosenhek, Jackie (October 2011). "Doctors of the Black Death". Doctor's Review. Rosenhek, Jackie (October 2011). "Doctors of the Black Death". Doctor's Review. Archivedfrom the original on 2014-05-06. Retrieved 2014-05-06.

Gottfried, Robert S. (1983). The Black Death: natural and human disaster in medieval Europe. Simon & Schuster. pp. 126–28.

Answers

Chapter 1: Greek and Latin

eye, dentistry, straight, child, paediatrics, radiation, childbirth, female, diseases, skin, tumors, urine, nervous, primary, hospitality, elderly.

Chapter 2: Equipment

stethoscope, sphygmomanometer, thermometer, infrared, pulse oximeter, fingertip, glucometer, ECG, cardiac, IV, nebulizer, defibrillator, patient monitoring, syringes, otoscope, ophthalmoscope, medical scales, medical, nitrile, Nitrile.

Chapter 3: Brain Anatomy

Cerebrum, frontal, Broca, parietal, somatosensory, occipital, temporal, temporal, brainstem, midbrain, cerebellum, ataxia, parietal, temporal, frontal.

Chapter 4: Neurons and Glial Cells

cell bodies, axons, astrocytes, White, 1,370, 1,200, language, neurons, fact, intuitive, Prefrontal, pleasant

Chapter 5: Grey Matter

sex, sloping, supraorbital, rounded, eye, 40, testosterone, type 2, atherosclerosis, knee, testosterone, cardiovascular, ACL, Q, lower, torque, heart, menopause, medicine, nutrition, mitigate, physical.

Chapter 6: Physiology

sex, sloping, supraorbital, rounded, eye, 40, testosterone, type 2, atherosclerosis, knee, testosterone, cardiovascular, ACL, Q, lower, torque, heart, menopause, medicine, nutrition, mitigate, physical.

Chapter 7: Wound Care

sharp, straight, jagged, irregular, outer, pointed, deep, enters, internal, bruise, blood, bruise, elevated, direct, immobilized, sucking, inhibiting, rabid, toxins.

Chapter 8: Immunology

self, foreign, Autoimmune, Innate, Adaptive, Cytokines, Cytotoxins, antibodies, endogenously, messengers, allergic, Natural killer, Cytokines.

Chapter 9: Pulmonary

Nasal, larynx, bronchi, alveoli, inhalation, exhalation, diaphragm/intercostal, oxygen, pulmonary

Chapter 10: Digestive

mouth, saliva, peristalsis, stomach, hydrochloric, pepsin, small, liver, pancreas, colon, water, rectum, anus, ingestion, Chemical, reflux, syndrome.

Chapter 11: Cardio1

cardiovascular, blood, thoracic, pump, atria, ventricles, mitral, cardiac, relaxation, Arteries, elastic, Veins, valves, nutrients, platelets, left, right, arrhythmias.

Chapter 12: Cardio 2

circulatory, blood, atria, ventricles, oxygen, oxygen, gases, Hypertension, Coronary, failure, Arrhythmias, stroke, Peripheral, Deep, legs, Pulmonary.

Chapter 13: Lymphatic

lymphatic, fluid, lymph, Lymph, spleen, thymus, digestive, Lymphedema, Lymphadenopathy, Lymphangitis, Lymphoma, Tonsillitis, Adenoiditis, physical.

Chapter 14: Quarantine

quarantine, Latin, Italian, red, Quarantine, Isolation, outbreak, epidemic, pandemic, humans, solid-front, treatments, cures, Patient, hemorrhagic, protective, personnel, environment

Chapter 15: Childhood development

Piaget, Vygotsky, childhood, four, Sensorimotor, object, Concrete, conservation, social, cultural, Zone, skilled, language, speech, solitary, social, learning, readiness, teacher, language.

Chapter 16: Paediatric Disease

Supportive, varicella, vaccination/immunization, rubella, phototherapy, clean, dry, vitamin A, chicken pox, rubella, lights, jaundice, regularly, antifungal

Chapter 17: Geriatric Disease

Hypertension/heart disease, stroke, diet, arthritis, physical, medications, osteoporosis, memory, blood sugar, diet, cough, psychotherapy, interventions, incontinence, bladder, central, supplements, medications, hearing, implants, vitamin, low

Chapter 18: Hospice

Comfort, palliative, social, pain, challenges, religion, practical, palliative, home, directives, bereavement, care

Chapter 19: Ethics

Moral, Hippocratic, Nightingale, regulations, patient, confidentiality, consent, Aktion, human, Nuremberg, ethical, malpractice, cultural, Nightingale, integrity

Chapter 20: Teamwork

Patient safety, various teams, a single team, set goals, roles, communication, respect, conflict, supportive, adaptable, job satisfaction, workplace happiness, patient outcomes, cost, transparency, open, professional development training, example

Made in United States
Cleveland, OH
05 November 2026

47667160R00129